CRAM SESSION IN

Manual Muscle Testing

A Handbook for Students & Clinicians

LYNN VAN OST

CRAM SESSION IN
Manual Muscle Testing
A Handbook for Students & Clinicians

LYNN VAN OST

LYNN VAN OST, MEd, RN, PT, ATC
University Orthopedic Associates
Somerset, New Jersey

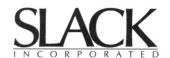

SLACK
INCORPORATED

www.slackbooks.com

ISBN: 978-1-55642-997-2

The procedures and practices described in this publication should be implemented in a manner consistent with the professional standards set for the circumstances that apply in each specific situation. Every effort has been made to confirm the accuracy of the information presented and to correctly relate generally accepted practices. The authors, editors, and publisher cannot accept responsibility for errors or exclusions or for the outcome of the material presented herein. There is no expressed or implied warranty of this book or information imparted by it. Care has been taken to ensure that drug selection and dosages are in accordance with currently accepted/recommended practice. Off-label uses of drugs may be discussed. Due to continuing research, changes in government policy and regulations, and various effects of drug reactions and interactions, it is recommended that the reader carefully review all materials and literature provided for each drug, especially those that are new or not frequently used. Some drugs or devices in this publication have clearance for use in a restricted research setting by the Food and Drug and Administration or FDA. Each professional should determine the FDA status of any drug or device prior to use in their practice. Any review or mention of specific companies or products is not intended as an endorsement by the author or publisher.

SLACK Incorporated uses a review process to evaluate submitted material. Prior to publication, educators or clinicians provide important feedback on the content that we publish. We welcome feedback on this work.

Published by: SLACK Incorporated
                  6900 Grove Road
                  Thorofare, NJ 08086 USA
                  Telephone: 856-848-1000
                  Fax: 856-848-6091
                  www.slackbooks.com

Contact SLACK Incorporated for more information about other books in this field or about the availability of our books from distributors outside the United States.

Van Ost, Lynn.
  Cram session in manual muscle testing : a handbook for students & clinicians / Lynn Van Ost.
     p. ; cm.
Includes bibliographical references and index.
ISBN 978-1-55642-997-2 (alk. paper)
I. Title.
[DNLM: 1. Muscle Strength--physiology. 2. Muscle Weakness--diagnosis. 3. Muscles--physiology. 4. Range of Motion, Articular--physiology. WE 500]

   616.7'40754--dc23

                          2011046551

Printed in the United States of America.

Last digit is print number: 10   9   8   7   6   5   4   3   2   1

DEDICATION

To my dad, William C. Van Ost, MD, who always encouraged me to continue to grab for the next rung on the ladder.

CONTENTS

ACKNOWLEDGMENTS

I would like to thank the many individuals who assisted me in order to make this project possible. First and foremost, those at SLACK Incorporated: John Bond, April Billick, and Michelle Gatt, whose support has been endless. I am grateful for your professionalism and friendship.

I am especially grateful to Andy Overman, who spent many hours being photographed as the model for this book. Thank you so much for your patience and flexibility during our photo sessions. This book could not have been produced without your help. I also want to thank Karen Manfre and Jenine LaFevere for once again serving as the examiners in the photographs. I really appreciated you going out of your way to help me complete this project.

Finally, I want to thank Billy Manfre for supporting me through many hours of typing and editing on the computer. The process was much easier with you by my side.

ABOUT THE AUTHOR

Lynn Van Ost, MEd, RN, PT, ATC graduated in 1982 with a bachelor's degree in nursing from West Chester State College, West Chester, PA; National Athletic Trainers' Association Board of Certification (NATABOC) certified in athletic training in 1984; graduated in 1987 from Temple University, Philadelphia, PA, with a master's degree in sports medicine/athletic training; and received a second bachelor's degree in physical therapy in 1988 from Temple. In addition to treating the general orthopedic population as a physical therapist, she has worked with both amateur and professional athletes and has more than 11 years of experience as an athletic trainer working with Olympic-level elite athletes at numerous international events, including the 1992 and 1996 Summer Olympic games. She currently works as the Director of Physical Therapy for University Orthopedic Associates in Somerset, New Jersey.

PREFACE

There are many textbooks on the market dedicated either wholly or in part to the topic of manual muscle testing; however, there are few books available that serve as a stand-alone quick reference for the clinician or student. The idea behind this manual was born from the need for a reference that would supply the clinician or student with a snapshot view of the basics of manual muscle testing. This manual was not designed or intended as a teaching tool or as an introductory text on the subject of manual muscle testing. It does not contain information on the theories of manual muscle testing; other textbooks cover those areas sufficiently. This book is intended as a simple, user-friendly reference for the experienced clinician or student.

Although this manual was primarily intended for use by physical therapists, athletic trainers, and occupational therapists, its use is not limited to those specialties. It could easily find a home on the office shelf of any health care provider who performs musculoskeletal examinations.

The text is organized by body region in a "head-to-toe" format to make it easier and more efficient to locate a specific test. Each region is subdivided into the specific movement to be tested, active range of motion, the prime movers of the movement, the secondary movers, the anti-gravity subject position, gravity minimized subject position, stabilization and grades, substitutions for the movement, and points of interest for that particular muscle group. There are also over 200 photographs that illustrate testing in both the anti-gravity and gravity minimized positions. Finally, there are 4 appendices that describe manual muscle testing grading, general procedures for testing, terminology, and factors that may cause inaccurate muscle testing.

It is the hope of the author that the material has been presented in a user-friendly format, making the task of manual muscle testing a bit easier to accomplish in the clinical setting.

SECTION I

Neck / Upper Extremities

Van Ost, L.
Cram Session in Manual Muscle Testing:
A Handbook for Students & Clinicians (pp. 1-98)
© 2012 SLACK Incorporated

NECK

FLEXION

ACTIVE RANGE OF MOTION

- 0 to 45 degrees with a goniometer
- 1.0 to 4.3 cm with a tape measure

PRIME MOVERS

- Sternocleidomastoid (SCM)

  □ Origin

    o Sternal head: Cranial aspect of the ventral surface of the manubrium.

    o Clavicular head: Superior border and anterior surface of the medial one third of the clavicle.

  □ Insertion: Lateral surface of the mastoid process and lateral half of the superior nuchal line of the occipital bone.

  □ Innervation: Spinal accessory nerve (C2 and C3 anterior rami).

  □ Other actions: Lateral flexion (to the same side) and rotation (to the opposite side) of the neck/head.

  □ Palpation site: Anterolateral aspect of the neck.

SECONDARY MOVERS

- Rectus capitits anterior
- Rectus capitis lateralis
- Suprahyoid
- Infrahyoid
- Platysma
- Scalenes
- Longus capitis
- Longus colli

ANTI-GRAVITY

Subject position: Supine on a table.

Stabilization: Weight of the trunk and clinician's hand on the thorax.

- Grades 5/5 to +3/5: See Figure 1-1.

Figure 1-1. Resistance is applied to the anterior forehead.

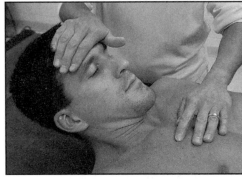

SUBJECT DIRECTIVE: *"Lift your head up off the table. Do not lift your shoulders up and do not let me push your head down."*

*The 2 SCM muscles may be tested individually by rotation of the head to one side with neck flexion.

- Grade 3/5: See Figure 1-2.

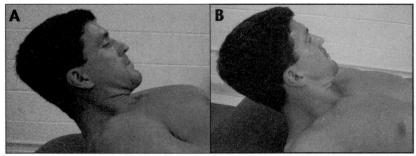

Figure 1-2. (A) The subject flexes the neck through the maximal range of motion without resistance. (B) Cervical rotation with flexion.

- Grades −3/5 to +2/5: See Figure 1-3.

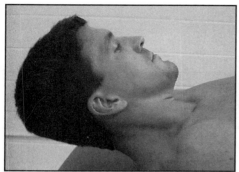

Figure 1-3. The subject flexes the neck through partial range of motion.

GRAVITY MINIMIZED

Subject position: Sidelying with the head supported on a smooth surface.

Stabilization: The clinician stabilizes the lower thorax.

- Grades 2/5 to −2/5: See Figure 1-4A.

- Grade 2/5: See Figure 1-4B.

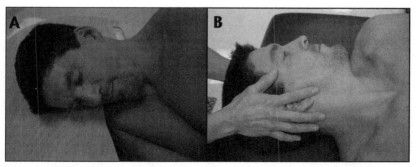

Figure 1-4. (A) The subject flexes the neck through the maximal range of motion. (B) As an option, the subject may be asked to rotate the head to one side and then to the other.

- Grades 1/5 to 0/5: See Figure 1-5.

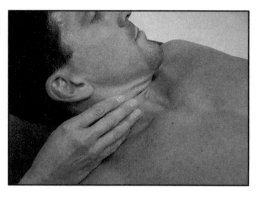

Figure 1-5. The sternocleidomastoid muscles are palpated on the sides of the neck while the subject attempts to flex.

Substitutions: The corners of the subject's mouth may be pulled down if the platysma contracts.

Points of interest: Torticollis may result if the sternocleidomastoid becomes dystonic.

EXTENSION

ACTIVE RANGE OF MOTION

- 0 to 45 degrees

PRIME MOVERS

- Splenius capitis

    □ Origin: Caudal half of the ligamentum nuchae and spinous processes of C7 and T1 to T4 vertebrae.

    □ Insertion: Occipital bone just inferior to the lateral one third of the superior nuchal line into the mastoid process of the temporal bone.

    □ Innervation: Lateral branches of the dorsal primary cervical nerves.

    □ Other actions: Slight rotation and lateral flexion of the head.

    □ Palpation site: Under the lateral borders of the upper trapezius.

- Semispinalis capitis

    □ Origin: Tips of the transverse processes of the C7 and T1 to T7 vertebrae.

    □ Insertion: Between the superior and inferior nuchal lines of the occipital bone.

- ☐ Innervation: Dorsal primary divisions of the cervical nerves.

- ☐ Other actions: Unilaterally: Rotation of the spine to the opposite side.

- ☐ Palpation site: Under the lateral borders of the upper trapezius.

- Cervicis muscles

  - ☐ Origin: Spinous processes of the T3 to T6 vertebrae.

  - ☐ Insertion: Posterior tubercles of C1 to C3.

  - ☐ Innervation: Dorsal primary branch of the spinal nerves.

  - ☐ Other actions: Unilaterally: Lateral flexion and rotation of the head.

  - ☐ Palpation site: Under the lateral borders of the upper trapezius.

SECONDARY MOVERS

- Upper trapezius

ANTI-GRAVITY

Subject position: Prone on a table.

Stabilization: Weight of the trunk and the clinician's hand on the upper thoracic area and scapulae.

- Grades 5/5 to +3/5: See Figure 1-6.

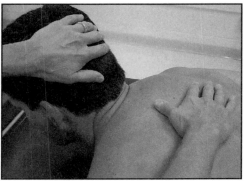

Figure 1-6. Resistance is applied to the occiput.

SUBJECT DIRECTIVE: *"Lift your head up toward the ceiling. Do not let me push your head down."*

- Grade 3/5: See Figure 1-7.

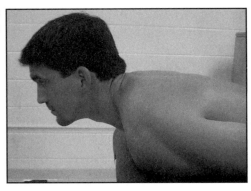

Figure 1-7. The subject extends the neck through the maximal range of motion without resistance.

- Grades −3/5 to +2/5: See Figure 1-8.

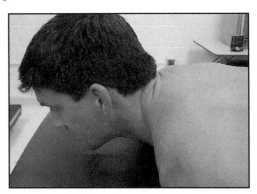

Figure 1-8. The subject extends the neck through partial range of motion.

GRAVITY MINIMIZED

Subject position: Sidelying with the head supported on a smooth surface.

Stabilization: Weight of the trunk on the table.

- Grades 2/5 to –2/5: See Figure 1-9.

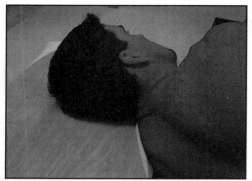

Figure 1-9. The subject extends the neck through the maximal range of motion.

- Grades 1/5 to 0/5: See Figure 1-10.

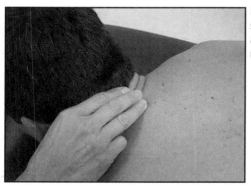

Figure 1-10. The splenius capitis, semispinalis capitis, and cervicis muscles are palpated on the posterior aspect of the neck while the subject tries to extend.

Substitutions: The subject may try to use the back muscles to lift the upper trunk from the table.

Points of interest: Tasks such as reaching overhead into a high cabinet, the top shelf in a closet, or drinking out of a cup require the contraction of the the cervical extensors at the end of the range of motion.

SCAPULA

ABDUCTION/UPWARD ROTATION

ACTIVE RANGE OF MOTION

- Right and left sides should be symmetrical when measured with a tape measure.

PRIME MOVERS

- Serratus anterior

  □ Origin: Anterior surfaces of ribs 1 through 9.

  □ Insertion: Anterior aspect of the medial border of the scapula from superior to inferior angle.

  □ Innervation: Long thoracic nerve (C5 to C7).

  □ Other actions: Stabilizes the scapula against the chest wall.

  □ Palpation site: Along the midaxillary line adjacent to the inferior angle of the scapula.

SECONDARY MOVERS

- Pectoralis minor

ANTI-GRAVITY

Subject position: Supine with the shoulder flexed to 90 degrees and the elbow in extension.

Stabilization: Weight of the trunk against the table.

- Grades 5/5 to +3/5: See Figure 1-11.

Figure 1-11. Resistance is given in a downward/inward direction by grasping the forearm and elbow.

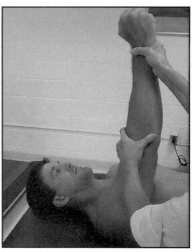

SUBJECT DIRECTIVE: *"Punch up toward the ceiling and resist as I push down."*

- Grades 3/5 to + 2/5: See Figure 1-12.

Figure 1-12. The subject moves the arm upward from a resting position on the table without resistance.

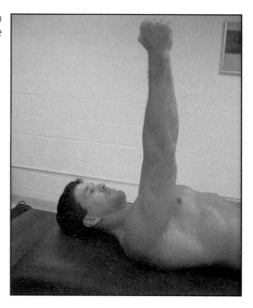

GRAVITY MINIMIZED

Subject position: Sitting with the upper arm resting on a table in 90 degrees of shoulder flexion and with the elbow extended.

Stabilization: Clinician stabilizes the thorax to prevent rotation or forward movement.

- Grades 2/5 to −2/5: See Figure 1-13.

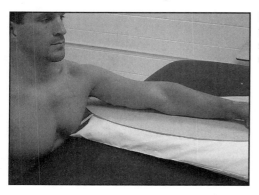

Figure 1-13. The subject moves the arm forward 2 to 3 inches by abducting the scapula through the maximal range of motion.

- Grades 1/5 to 0/5: See Figure 1-14.

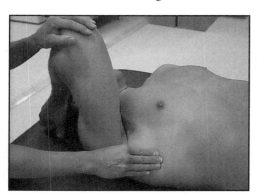

Figure 1-14. The serratus anterior is palpated along the midaxillary line adjacent to the inferior angle of the scapula as the subject attempts to abduct the scapula against light resistance.

Points of interest: Weakness of the serratus anterior causes "winging" of the scapula, which is most evident when standing and pushing against a wall. It is the strongest abductor of the scapula and weakness of this muscle makes it difficult to flex or abduct the shoulder.

ADDUCTION/DOWNWARD ROTATION

ACTIVE RANGE OF MOTION

■ Right and left sides should be symmetrical when measured with a tape measure.

PRIME MOVERS

■ Rhomboid major

□ Origin: Spinous processes of T2 to T5.

□ Insertion: Medial border of the scapula between the spine and inferior angle.

□ Innervation: Dorsal scapular nerve (C5).

□ Other actions: Scapular stabilization.

□ Palpation site: With the subject's hand behind his or her lumbar spine, palpate under and along the medial border of the scapula.

■ Rhomboid minor

□ Origin: Spinous processes of C7 and T1.

□ Insertion: The medial border of the scapula at the level of the spine of the scapula.

□ Innervation: Dorsal scapular nerve (C5).

□ Other actions: Scapular stabilization.

□ Palpation site: With the subject's hand behind his or her lumbar spine, palpate under and along the medial border of the scapula.

SECONDARY MOVERS

■ Middle trapezius

■ Levator scapulae

ANTI-GRAVITY

Subject position: Prone with the tested upper extremity behind the back with the hand resting on the lumbar spine. The head is rotated to the opposite side.

Stabilization: The clinician stabilizes the thorax on the opposite side.

- Grades 5/5 to +3/5: See Figure 1-15.

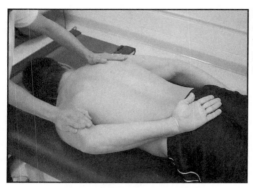

Figure 1-15. As the subject lifts his hand off the back, resistance is applied above the elbow in a down and out direction, pushing the scapula into abduction and upward rotation.

SUBJECT DIRECTIVE: *"Lift your hand up toward the ceiling and do not let me push your arm down."*

- Grade 3/5: See Figure 1-16.

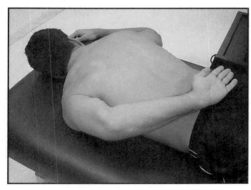

Figure 1-16. The subject lifts his hand off the back as the scapula is adducted through the maximal range of motion.

GRAVITY MINIMIZED

Subject position: Sitting with the tested arm internally rotated and adducted behind the lumbar spine.

Stabilization: The clinician stabilizes the anterior/posterior trunk, if necessary, to prevent flexion or rotation.

- Grades 2/5 to −2/5: See Figure 1-17.

Figure 1-17. The subject attempts to adduct the scapula through the range of motion.

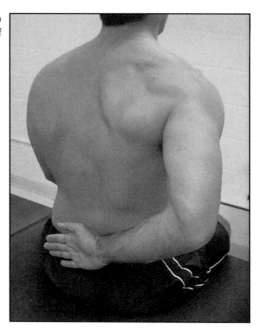

- Grades 1/5 to 0/5: See Figure 1-18.

Figure 1-18. The rhomboids may be palpated under and along the medial border of the scapula as the subject attempts to adduct the scapula.

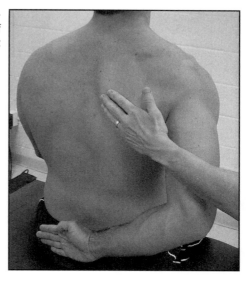

Substitutions: The latissimus dorsi and teres major may cause the shoulder to adduct and extend the shoulder without scapular rotation. The subject may use the wrist extensors to lift the upper extremity off the lower back without scapular movement.

Points of interest: Weakness of the rhomboids may cause medial scapular winging and decreased strength of shoulder adduction and extension due to loss of scapular stabilization.

ELEVATION

PRIME MOVERS

- Upper trapezius

  - □ Origin: External occipital protuberance, medial third superior nuchal line, and the ligamentum nuchae.

  - □ Insertion: Posterior border of the lateral third of the clavicle and acromion process.

  - □ Innervation: Spinal accessory nerve (CN XI).

  - □ Other actions: Lateral rotation of the scapula.

  - □ Palpation site: The superior and posterior surface of the shoulders.

- Levator scapulae

  - □ Origin: Transverse processes of C1 to C4.

  - □ Insertion: Medial border of the scapula at the level of the scapular superior angle.

  - □ Innervation: Dorsal scapular nerve (C5) and C3, C4.

  - □ Other actions: Medial rotation of the scapula and scapular stabilization.

  - □ Palpation site: Deep to the upper trapezius in the angle formed by the upper trapezius and sternocleidomastoid muscles.

SECONDARY MOVERS

- Rhomboids major and minor

ANTI-GRAVITY

Subject position: Sitting in a chair or on a table with the arms hanging by the sides.

Stabilization: Achieved through subject compliance.

- Grades 5/5 to +3/5: See Figure 1-19.

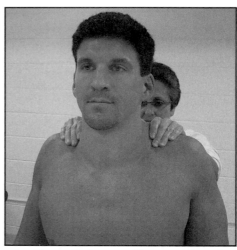

Figure 1-19. Resistance is applied symmetrically in a downward direction on top of the shoulders.

SUBJECT DIRECTIVE: *"Raise your shoulders as high as possible toward the ceiling and hold while I try to push them down."*

- Grades 3/5 to +2/5: See Figure 1-20.

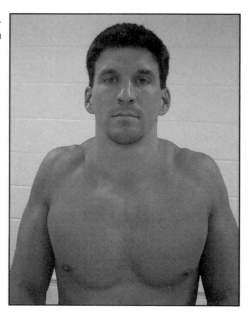

Figure 1-20. The subject elevates the shoulders through the maximal range of motion without resistance.

GRAVITY MINIMIZED

Subject position: Supine or prone on a table with the arms by the sides.

Stabilization: Weight of the trunk on the table.

- Grades 2/5 to –2/5: See Figure 1-21.

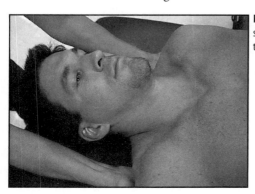

Figure 1-21. As the clinician supports the shoulders, the subject elevates the shoulders toward the ears.

- Grades 1/5 to 0/5: See Figure 1-22.

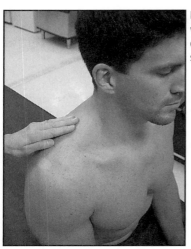

Figure 1-22. The upper trapezius is palpated to the cervical vertebrae and its insertion at the superior/posterior aspect of the distal clavicle as the subject attempts to elevate the shoulders.

Points of interest: Weakness of the upper trapezius may cause lateral winging of the scapula, which is most obvious when attempting to abduct the shoulder. Weakness of the upper trapezius also causes difficulty when trying to abduct or flex the upper extremity above shoulder height.

ADDUCTION

ACTIVE RANGE OF MOTION

- Right and left sides should be symmetrical when measured with a tape measure.

PRIME MOVERS

- Middle trapezius

  □ Origin: Inferior aspect of the ligamentum nuchae, spinous processes of C7 to T5.

  □ Insertion: Medial aspect of the acromion process and superior lip of the spine of the scapula.

  □ Innervation: Spinal accessory nerve (CN XI).

  □ Other actions: None.

  □ Palpation site: Medial border of the scapula near the root of the spine.

- Rhomboid major

  □ Origin: Spinous processes of T2 to T5.

  □ Insertion: Medial border of the scapula between the spine and inferior angle.

  □ Innervation: Dorsal scapular nerve (C5).

  □ Other actions: Scapular stabilization.

  □ Palpation site: With the subject's hand behind his or her lumbar spine, palpate under and along the medial border of the scapula.

- Rhomboid minor

  □ Origin: Spinous processes of C7 to T1.

  □ Insertion: The medial border of the scapula at the level of the spine of the scapula.

  □ Innervation: Dorsal scapular nerve (C5).

  □ Other actions: Scapular stabilization.

  □ Palpation site: With the subject's hand behind his or her lumbar spine, palpate under and along the medial border of the scapula.

SECONDARY MOVERS

- Upper and lower trapezius

ANTI-GRAVITY

Subject position: Prone on a table with the shoulder in 90 degrees of abduction and with the elbow flexed to 90 degrees, the forearm hanging freely over the edge of a table.

Stabilization: Weight of the trunk on the table. The clinician stabilizes the contralateral thorax.

- Grades 5/5 to +3/5: See Figure 1-23.

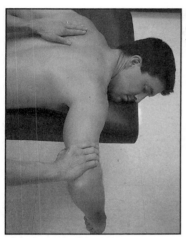

Figure 1-23. Resistance is applied just proximal to the elbow toward the floor as the subject horizontally abducts the shoulder and adducts the scapula.

SUBJECT DIRECTIVE: *"Squeeze your shoulder blades together and push your arm up into my hand and hold it. Do not let me push your arm down."*

- Grades 3/5 to +2/5: See Figure 1-24.

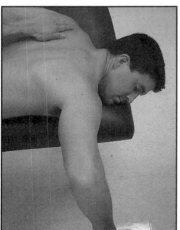

Figure 1-24. The subject raises his arm toward the ceiling while adducting the scapula through the available range of motion without resistance.

GRAVITY MINIMIZED

Subject position: Sitting with the arm resting on a table with the shoulder abducted to 90 degrees and the elbow flexed to 90 degrees.

Stabilization: The clinician stabilizes the contralateral thorax.

- Grades 2/5 to –2/5: See Figure 1-25.

Figure 1-25. The subject horizontally abducts the shoulder and adducts the scapula through the available range of motion.

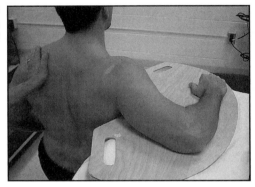

- Grades 1/5 to 0/5: See Figure 1-26.

Figure 1-26. The middle trapezius is palpated along the medial border of the scapula between thoracic vertebrae T1 to T5 and near the root of the spine of the scapula as the subject attempts to horizontally abduct the shoulder.

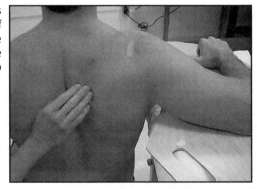

Substitutions: The posterior deltoid may cause horizontal abduction of the shoulder without scapular adduction. The lower trapezius may cause depression to occur and the rhomboids may slightly elevate and downwardly rotate the scapula.

DEPRESSION/ADDUCTION

PRIME MOVERS

- Lower trapezius

- [ ] Origin: Spinous processes of T6 to T12.

- [ ] Insertion: The root and inferiorly on the spine of the scapula.

- [ ] Innervation: Spinal accessory nerve (CN XI).

- [ ] Other actions: None.

- [ ] Palpation site: Medial to the root of the spine and the medial border of the scapula.

SECONDARY MOVERS

- Middle trapezius

- Pectoralis minor

- Latissimus dorsi

- Pectoralis major

- Pectoralis minor

ANTI-GRAVITY

Subject position: Prone with the head rotated to the same side and tested shoulder in approximately 130 degrees of abduction and with the elbow in extension.

Stabilization: The clinician stabilizes the contralateral thorax.

- Grades 5/5 to +3/5: See Figure 1-27.

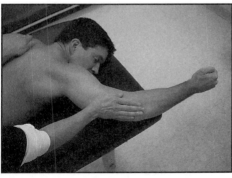

Figure 1-27. Resistance is applied just proximal to the elbow joint directed down toward the floor.

SUBJECT DIRECTIVE: *"Raise your arm up off the table as far as you can and hold it. Do not let me push it down."*

- Grade 3/5: See Figure 1-28.

Figure 1-28. The subject lifts the limb off the table without resistance.

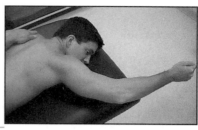

The upper extremity may be supported by the clinician into abduction if the deltoid is weak.

GRAVITY ELIMINATED/MINIMIZED

Subject position: Prone with the head rotated to the same side as the tested shoulder in approximately 130 degrees of abduction.

Stabilization: The clinician stabilizes the contralateral thorax.

- Grade 2/5: See Figure 1-29.

Figure 1-29. The subject is able to achieve full scapular movement with the tested limb supported.

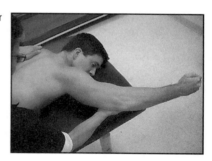

- Grades 1/5 to 0/5: See Figure 1-30.

Figure 1-30. The lower trapezius is palpated medial to the root of the spine and medial border of the scapula as the subject attempts to lift the arm off the table.

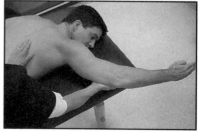

Substitutions: The subject may try to extend the trunk to give the appearance of scapular movement.

SHOULDER

FLEXION

ACTIVE RANGE OF MOTION
- 0 to 180 degrees

PRIME MOVERS
- Anterior deltoid
  - □ Origin: Anterior and superior lateral third of the clavicle.
  - □ Insertion: Deltoid tuberosity of the humerus.
  - □ Innervation: Axillary nerve (C5 to C6).
  - □ Other actions: Internally rotates and horizontally adducts the shoulder.
  - □ Palpation site: Inferior to the lateral third of the clavicle.
- Coracobrachialis (up to 90 degrees of shoulder flexion)
  - □ Origin: Coracoid process of the scapula.
  - □ Insertion: Medial surface of the midshaft of the humerus.
  - □ Innervation: Musculocutaneous nerve (C6 to C7).
  - □ Other actions: Scaption of the shoulder.
  - □ Palpation site: Deep into the upper middle third of the arm, in the axilla, under the inferior border of the pectoralis major muscle.

SECONDARY MOVERS
- Middle deltoid
- Pectoralis major
- Biceps brachii

ANTI-GRAVITY
Subject position: Sitting with the shoulder flexed to 90 degrees, palm facing down.

Stabilization: The clinician stabilizes the opposite scapula.

- Grades 5/5 to +3/5: See Figure 1-31.

Figure 1-31. Resistance is applied in a downward direction just proximal to the elbow joint.

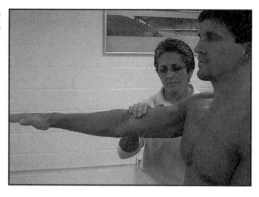

SUBJECT DIRECTIVE: *"Hold your arm up and do not let me push it down."*

- Grades 3/5: See Figure 1-32.

Figure 1-32. The subject flexes the shoulder to at least 90 degrees without resistance.

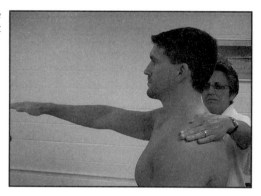

GRAVITY MINIMIZED

Subject position: Sidelying with the upper extremity supported on a smooth surface and in neutral rotation with the elbow in flexion.

Stabilization: The opposite shoulder is stabilized by the weight of the body against the table.

- Grades 2/5 to –2/5: See Figure 1-33.

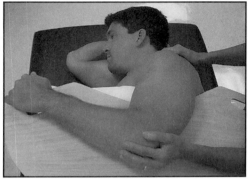

Figure 1-33. The subject flexes the shoulder through the maximal range of motion.

- Grades 1/5 to 0/5: See Figure 1-34.

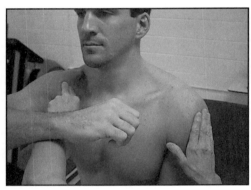

Figure 1-34. The anterior deltoid is palpated inferiorly to the lateral third of the clavicle. The coracobrachialis is palpated in the axilla along the inferior border of the pectoralis major muscle.
(Shown: Palpating the anterior deltoid.)

Substitutions: If the upper trapezius is activated, the scapula will elevate. Substitution by the pectoralis major will cause horizontal adduction. The subject may also externally rotate the shoulder to substitute with the biceps or lean back into trunk extension to give the appearance of shoulder flexion.

EXTENSION

ACTIVE RANGE OF MOTION

- 180 to 0 degrees

- 0 to 40/60 degrees (from neutral)

PRIME MOVERS

- Latissimus dorsi

  - Origin: Lumbar aponeurosis, spinous processes of T6 to T12, L1 to L5, and the sacral vertebrae.

  - Insertion: Medial lip of the intertubercular groove of the humerus.

  - Innervation: Thoracodorsal nerve (C6 to C8).

  - Other actions: Adducts and internally rotates the shoulder and assists with scapular depression.

  - Palpation site: Along the midaxillary line on the trunk.

- Teres major

  - Origin: Posterior surface of the inferior scapular angle.

  - Insertion: Crest of the lessor tubercle of the humerus.

  - Innervation: Lower subscapular nerve (C6).

  - Other actions: Adduction and internal rotation of the shoulder.

  - Palpation site: Lateral to the inferior angle of the scapula.

- Posterior deltoid

  - Origin: Inferior lip of the posterior border of the spine of the scapula.

  - Insertion: Deltoid tuberosity of the humerus.

  - Innervation: Axillary nerve (C5 to C6).

  - Other actions: External rotation and horizontal abduction of the shoulder.

  - Palpation site: Inferior and lateral to the spine of the scapula.

SECONDARY MOVERS

- Long head of the triceps brachii

ANTI-GRAVITY

Subject position: The subject should be prone with the arms at the sides and with the palm facing up toward the ceiling.

Stabilization: The weight of the thorax against the table.

- Grades 5/5 to +3/5: See Figure 1-35.

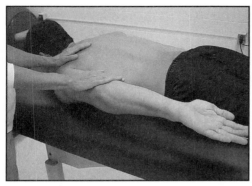

Figure 1-35. Resistance is applied at the elbow in a downward direction toward the floor.

SUBJECT DIRECTIVE: *"Lift your arm as high as you can toward the ceiling and hold it. Do not let me push it down."*

- Grade 3/5: See Figure 1-36.

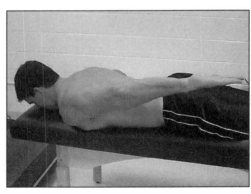

Figure 1-36. The subject lifts the arm up toward the ceiling through the maximal range of motion without resistance.

GRAVITY MINIMIZED

Subject position: Sidelying with the upper extremity supported on a smooth surface and in neutral rotation with the elbow in flexion.

Stabilization: The opposite shoulder is stabilized by the weight of the body against the table.

- Grades 2/5 to –2/5: See Figure 1-37.

Figure 1-37. The subject extends the shoulder through the maximal range of motion.

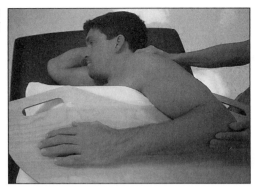

- Grades 1/5 to 0/5: See Figure 1-38.

Figure 1-38. The latissimus dorsi is palpated inferiorly and lateral to the inferior angle of the scapula on the side of the thoracic wall as the subject attempts to extend the shoulder. The teres major and posterior deltoid are palpable at the lateral border of the scapula just below the axilla and just superior to the axilla, respectively.
(Shown: palpating the latissimus dorsi)

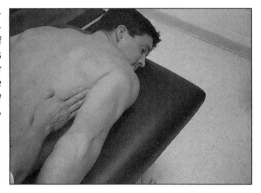

Substitutions: The subject may attempt to lift and rotate the trunk.

Points of interest: The latissimus dorsi is a powerful shoulder extensor and is active during forceful activities such as swimming, rowing/paddling, or chopping movements. It pulls the shoulder girdle down during any activity that requires the body to be pulled toward the arm as in crutch walking or rock climbing. The teres major is occasionally known as the "little latissimus" because it performs the same actions as the latissimus dorsi. In combination with the infraspinatus and teres minor, it pulls downward to help stabilize the head of the humerus during abduction.

ABDUCTION

ACTIVE RANGE OF MOTION

- 0 to 180 degrees

PRIME MOVERS

- Middle deltoid

  □ Origin: Superior/lateral surface of the acromion process of the scapula.

  □ Insertion: Deltoid tuberosity of the humerus.

  □ Innervation: Axillary nerve (C5 to C6).

  □ Other actions: Scaption.

  □ Palpation site: Lateral/inferior to the acromion process.

SECONDARY MOVERS

- Supraspinatus

ANTI-GRAVITY

Subject position: Sitting with the shoulder abducted to 90 degrees, palm down.

Stabilization: The clinician stabilizes the opposite shoulder.

- Grades 5/5 to +3/5: See Figure 1-39.

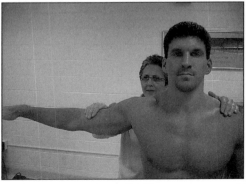

Figure 1-39. Resistance is applied just proximal to the elbow in a downward direction toward the floor.

SUBJECT DIRECTIVE: *"Hold your arm up and do not let me push it down."*

- Grade 3/5: See Figure 1-40.

Figure 1-40. The subject abducts the shoulder to at least 90 degrees without resistance.

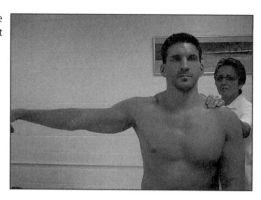

GRAVITY MINIMIZED

Subject position: Supine with the tested limb supported on a table.

Stabilization: Weight of the trunk on the table.

- Grades 2/5 to −2/5: See Figure 1-41.

Figure 1-41. The subject abducts the shoulder through the maximal range of motion.

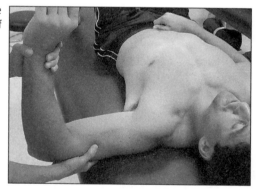

■ Grades 1/5 to 0/5: See Figure 1-42.

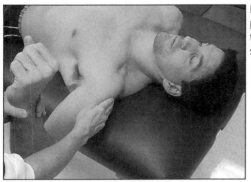

Figure 1-42. The middle deltoid is palpated lateral to the acrominon process on the superior aspect of the shoulder as the subject attempts to abduct the shoulder.

Substitutions: The subject may try to elevate the shoulder or laterally flex the trunk to give the illusion of shoulder abduction.

Points of interest: Although the deltoid is a strong abductor, it is the supraspinatus, not the deltoid, that initiates the movement because the angle of the pull of the middle deltoid is parallel to the shaft of the humerus when the upper extremity is positioned at the side.

HORIZONTAL ABDUCTION

ACTIVE RANGE OF MOTION
■ 0 to 45 degrees (from neutral)

PRIME MOVERS
■ Posterior deltoid

  □ Origin: Inferior lip of the posterior border of the spine of the scapula.

  □ Insertion: Deltoid tuberosity of the humerus.

  □ Innervation: Axillary nerve (C5 to C6).

  □ Other actions: Extends and externally rotates the shoulder.

  □ Palpation site: Inferior/lateral to the spine of the scapula.

SECONDARY MOVERS
■ Long head of the triceps brachii

ANTI-GRAVITY

Subject position: Prone with the shoulder in 90 degrees of abduction and with the forearm off the edge of the table with the elbow in flexion.

Stabilization: Weight of the trunk on the table.

- Grades 5/5 to +3/5: See Figure 1-43.

Figure 1-43. Resistance is applied just proximal to the elbow toward the floor.

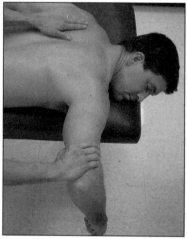

SUBJECT DIRECTIVE: *"Lift your elbow up toward the ceiling and hold it. Do not let me push it down."*

- Grades 3/5 to +2/5: See Figure 1-44.

Figure 1-44. The subject horizontally abducts the shoulder through the range of motion without resistance.

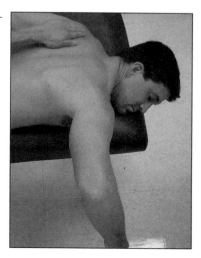

GRAVITY MINIMIZED

Subject position: Sitting with the arm supported on a table in 90 degrees of shoulder abduction and with the elbow in flexion.

Stabilization: The clinician stabilizes the scapula on the tested side.

■ Grades 2/5 to –2/5: See Figure 1-45.

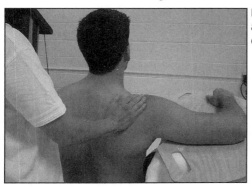

Figure 1-45. The subject horizontally abducts the shoulder through the range of motion.

■ Grades 1/5 to 0/5: See Figure 1-46.

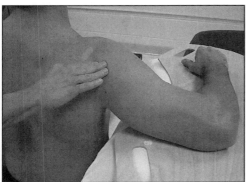

Figure 1-46. The posterior deltoid is palpated just below and lateral to the spine of the scapula as the subject attempts to horizontally abduct the shoulder.

Substitutions: The subject may extend the elbow when substituting with the triceps brachii or rotate the trunk during testing.

HORIZONTAL ADDUCTION

ACTIVE RANGE OF MOTION

■ 0 to 90 degrees (from neutral)

PRIME MOVERS

- Pectoralis major

  □ Origin:

    o Clavicular head: Anterior surface of the medial half of the clavicle.

    o Sternal head: Anterior surface of the sternum, the costal cartilages of the upper 6 pairs of ribs, and the aponeurosis of the obliquus externus abdominis.

  □ Insertion:

    o Clavicular head: Inferior crest of the greater tubercle of the humerus.

    o Sternal head: Superior crest of the greater tubercle of the humerus.

  □ Innervation: Medial pectoral nerve (C6 to T1).

  □ Other actions: Internal rotation of the shoulder. Clavicular head: flexion of the shoulder; sternal head: extension of the shoulder and anterior tilting of the scapula.

  □ Palpation site: Anterior axillary fold.

SECONDARY MOVERS

- Anterior deltoid
- Coracobrachialis
- Biceps brachii

ANTI-GRAVITY

Subject position: Supine with the shoulder in 90 degrees abduction and neutral rotation, elbow flexed to 90 degrees.

Stabilization: Weight of the trunk against the table.

- Grades 5/5 to +3/5: See Figure 1-47.

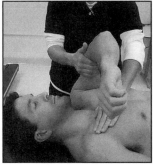

Figure 1-47. Resistance is applied to the anterior medial aspect of the arm just proximal to the elbow.

SUBJECT DIRECTIVE: *"Move your arm across your chest and do not let me pull it back."*

- Grade 3/5 to +2/5: See Figure 1-48.

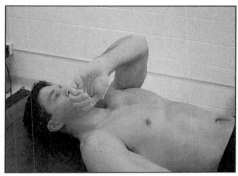

Figure 1-48. The subject horizontally adducts the shoulder through the maximal range of motion without resistance.

GRAVITY MINIMIZED

Subject position: Sitting with the shoulder supported on a table, abducted to 90 degrees, and in neutral rotation with the elbow flexed to 90 degrees.

Stabilization: The clinician stabilizes the contralateral shoulder.

- Grade 2/5 to –2/5: See Figure 1-49.

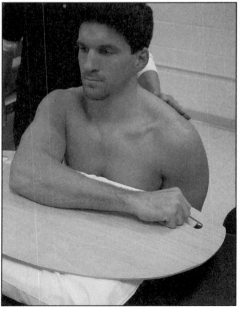

Figure 1-49. The subject horizontally adducts the shoulder through the range of motion.

- Grades 1/5 to 0/5: See Figure 1-50.

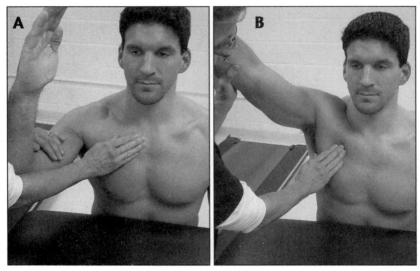

Figure 1-50. (A) The clavicular portion of the pectoralis major is palpated inferior to the medial end of the clavicle. (B) The sternal portion is palpated near the anterior axillary fold as the subject attempts to horizontally adduct and extend the shoulder.

Substitutions: The subject may attempt to rotate the trunk during testing.

Points of interest: The pectoralis major is important during supportive activites such as crutch walking or ambulating in parallel bars. The subject may be unable to touch the opposite shoulder or reach across the chest such as when trying to put a seat belt on if the pectoralis muscle is weak.

INTERNAL (MEDIAL) ROTATION

ACTIVE RANGE OF MOTION

- 0 to 90 degrees

PRIME MOVERS

- Subscapularis
  - □ Origin: Subscapular fossa.
  - □ Insertion: Lesser tubercle of the humerus.

- Innervation: Subscapular nerve (C5 to C6).

- Other actions: Slight adduction of the shoulder.

- Palpation site: On the lateral border of the costal surface of the scapula just deep to the latissimus dorsi muscle.

SECONDARY MOVERS

- Pectoralis major

- Teres major

- Latissimus dorsi

ANTI-GRAVITY/MINIMIZED

Subject position: Prone with the shoulder abducted to 90 degrees and the elbow flexed over the edge of the table. The head should be rotated to the tested side.

Stabilization: The clinician stabilizes the humerus and thorax.

- Grades 5/5 to +3/5: See Figure 1-51.

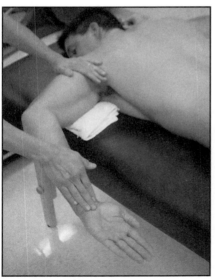

Figure 1-51. Resistance is applied to the flexor surface of the forearm just proximal to the wrist.

SUBJECT DIRECTIVE: *"Move your arm and hand up toward the ceiling and hold it. Do not let me push it down."*

- Grades 3/5 to +2/5: See Figure 1-52.

Figure 1-52. The subject internally rotates the shoulder through the maximal range of motion without resistance.

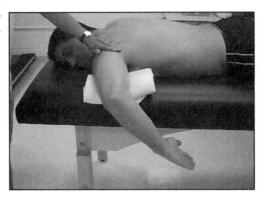

GRAVITY MINIMIZED

Subject position: Prone with the tested arm hanging freely over the edge of the table with the palm facing the table. The head should be rotated to the tested side.

Stabilization: The weight of the trunk on the table.

- Grades 2/5 to −2/5: See Figure 1-53.

Figure 1-53. The subject internally rotates the shoulder so that the palm faces away from the table. The thumb should initiate the movement.

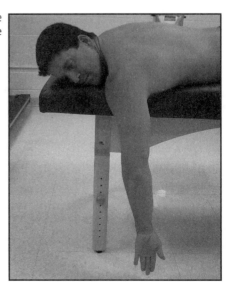

- Grades 1/5 to 0/5: See Figure 1-54.

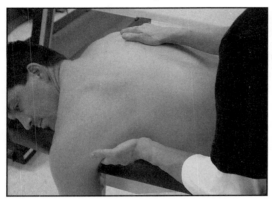

Figure 1-54. The subscapularis is palpated on the costal surface of the scapula just deep to the latissimus dorsi muscle as the subject attempts to internally rotate the shoulder.

Points of interest: The subscapularis is the only pure internal rotator of the shoulder and is most active when lifting the hand away from the back such as when tucking a shirt into a pair of pants or when hooking a bra.

EXTERNAL (LATERAL) ROTATION

ACTIVE RANGE OF MOTION

- 0 to 90 degrees

PRIME MOVERS

- Infraspinatus

  □ Origin: Infraspinatus fossa of the scapula.

  □ Insertion: Posterior on the greater tubercle of the humerus.

  □ Innervation: Suprascapular nerve (C5 to C6).

  □ Other actions: Slight extension of the shoulder.

  □ Palpation site: Inferior to the spine of the scapula.

- Teres minor

  □ Origin: Upper portion of the lateral border of the scapula.

  □ Insertion: Inferior on the posterior aspect of the greater tubercle of the humerus.

  □ Innervation: Axillary nerve (C5 to C6).

□ Other actions: Slight extension of the shoulder.

□ Palpation site: Lateral border of the scapula superior to the inferior angle of the scapula.

SECONDARY MOVERS

■ Posterior deltoid

ANTI-GRAVITY

Subject position: Prone with the shoulder abducted to 90 degrees and the elbow flexed over the edge of the table. The head should be rotated to the tested side.

Stabilization: The clinician stabilizes the humerus and thorax.

■ Grades 5/5 to +3/5: See Figure 1-55.

Figure 1-55. Resistance is applied to the extensor surface of the forearm just proximal to the wrist.

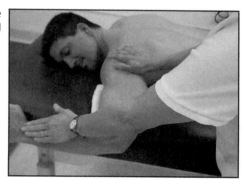

SUBJECT DIRECTIVE: *"Move your arm and the back of your hand up toward the ceiling and hold it. Do not let me push it down."*

■ Grades 3/5 to +2/5: See Figure 1-56.

Figure 1-56. The subject externally rotates the shoulder through the maximal range of motion without resistance.

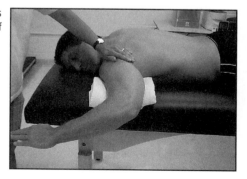

GRAVITY MINIMIZED

Subject position: Prone with the tested arm hanging freely over the edge of the table with the palm facing the table. The head should be rotated to the tested side.

Stabilization: The weight of the trunk on the table.

- Grades 2/5 to –2/5: See Figure 1-57.

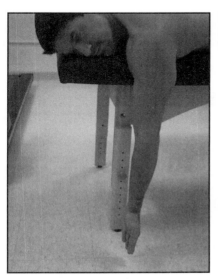

Figure 1-57. The subject externally rotates the shoulder so that the palm moves away from the table. The thumb should initiate the movement.

- Grades 1/5 to 0/5: See Figure 1-58.

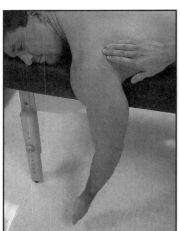

Figure 1-58. The infraspinatus is palpated inferiorly to the spine of the scapula and the teres minor is palpated along the lateral border of the scapula superior to the inferior angle of the scapula as the subject attempts to externally rotate the shoulder.
(Shown: Palpating the teres minor.)

Points of interest: The external rotators of the shoulder are functionally associated with the supinators of the forearm when the elbow is in extension, such as when using a screwdriver or installing a lightbulb into a socket on the ceiling.

SCAPTION

ACTIVE RANGE OF MOTION
- 0 to 180 degrees

PRIME MOVERS
- Supraspinatus
  - Origin: Supraspinatus fossa of the scapula.
  - Insertion: Superior surface of the greater tubercle of the humerus.
  - Innervation: Suprascapular nerve (C4 to C6).
  - Other actions: Abduction of the shoulder.
  - Palpation site: Above the spine of the scapula with the shoulder in approximately 30 degrees of shoulder flexion in the sagittal plane from the frontal plane.
- Anterior deltoid
  - Origin: Anterior and superior surface of the lateral third of the clavicle.
  - Insertion: Deltoid tuberosity of the humerus.
  - Innervation: Axillary nerve (C5 to C6).
  - Other actions: Flexion, internal rotation, and horizontal adduction of the shoulder.
  - Palpation site: Inferior to the lateral third of the clavicle.
- Middle deltoid
  - Origin: Superior lateral surface of the acromion process of the scapula.
  - Insertion: Deltoid tuberosity of the humerus.
  - Innervation: Axillary nerve (C5 to C6).
  - Other actions: Abduction of the shoulder to 90 degrees.
  - Palpation site: Lateral and inferior to the acromion process.

SECONDARY MOVERS

- None

ANTI-GRAVITY

Subject position: Sitting with the arm elevated approximately 30 degrees of shoulder flexion from the sagittal plane into the frontal plane. The thumb should point up to the ceiling.

Stabilization: The clinician stabilizes the opposite shoulder.

- Grades 5/5 to +3/5: See Figure 1-59.

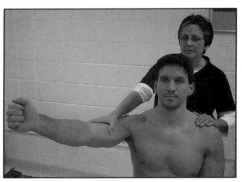

Figure 1-59. Resistance is applied just proximal to the elbow joint downward toward the floor.

SUBJECT DIRECTIVE: *"Lift your arm halfway between in front of and to the side of you and hold it. Do not let me push it down."*

- Grades 3/5 to +2/5: See Figure 1-60.

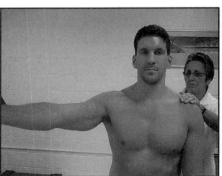

Figure 1-60. The subject moves the arm into scaption through the maximal range of motion.

GRAVITY MINIMIZED

Subject position: Sitting with the arms by the subject's sides.

Stabilization: The clinician stabilizes the opposite shoulder.

- Grades 2/5 to –2/5: See Figure 1-61.

Figure 1-61. The subject moves the arm through partial range of motion.

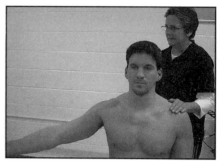

- Grades 1/5 to 0/5: See Figure 1-62.

Figure 1-62. The anterior deltoid is palpated inferiorly to the lateral third of the clavicle as the subject attempts to perform shoulder scaption. The supraspinatus is palpated superior to the spine of the scapula, with the shoulder in the plane of the scapula: approximately 30 degrees into the sagittal plane from the frontal plane.
(Shown: palpating the anterior deltoid)

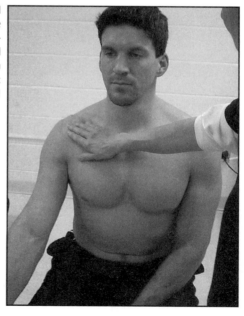

Points of interest: The supraspinatus is the muscle most often involved in shoulder "impingement syndrome." It is the major initiator of the first 15 degrees of humeral abduction and serves as a stabilizer for this motion.

ELBOW

FLEXION

ACTIVE RANGE OF MOTION

- 0 to 145 degrees

PRIME MOVERS

- Biceps brachii

  □ Origin:

    o Short head: Apex of the coracoid process.

    o Long head: Supraglenoid tuberosity at the superior margin of the glenoid.

  □ Insertion: Radial tuberosity and bicipital aponeurosis.

  □ Innervation: Musculocutaneous nerve (C6).

  □ Other actions: Forearm supination and shoulder flexion.

  □ Palpation site: With the forearm supinated, the belly of the muscle is palpated anteriorly or in the cubital fossa for the tendinous insertion.

- Brachialis

  □ Origin: Distal half of the anterior aspect of the humeral shaft.

  □ Insertion: Ulnar tuberosity and the anterior surface of the corocoid process.

  □ Innervation: Musculocutaneous and radial nerves (C6).

  □ Other actions: None.

  □ Palpation site: With the forearm pronated, palpate lateral/medial and deep to the biceps tendon just proximal to the cubital fossa.

- Brachioradialis

  □ Origin: Proximal two thirds of the lateral supracondylar ridge of the humerus.

  □ Insertion: Base of the styloid process of the radius.

  □ Innervation: Radial nerve (C6 to C7).

  □ Other actions: None.

☐ Palpation site: With the forearm midway between pronation and supination and with the elbow flexed to 90 degrees, palpate just lateral to the biceps tendon at the level of or proximal to the elbow joint.

SECONDARY MOVERS

- Pronator teres

- Extensor carpi radialis longus

- Flexor carpi radialis

- Flexor carpi ulnaris

ANTI-GRAVITY

Subject position: Sitting, with the elbow flexed to 90 degrees and the forearm supinated (biceps brachii), pronated (brachialis), or in neutral (brachioradialis), depending on which muscle is being tested. General elbow flexion is tested with the forearm in supination.

Stabilization: The clinician stabilizes the upper arm against the trunk.

- Grades 5/5 to +3/5: See Figure 1-63.

Figure 1-63. Resistance is applied on the anterior forearm just proximal to the wrist.

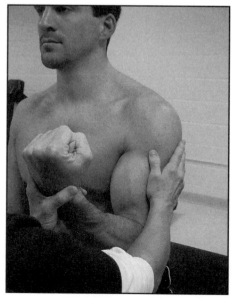

SUBJECT DIRECTIVE: *"Bend your elbow up. Do not let me pull your arm down."*

- Grades 3/5 to +2/5: See Figure 1-64.

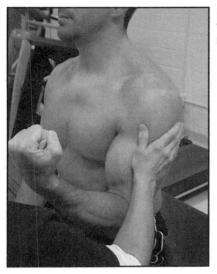

Figure 1-64. The subject flexes the elbow through the maximal available range of motion without resistance.

GRAVITY MINIMIZED

Subject position: Sitting, with the upper extremity resting on a smooth surface. The shoulder should be in 90 degrees of abduction with the elbow in maximal extension and the forearm in neutral rotation.

Stabilization: The clinician stabilizes the upper arm against the testing surface.

- Grades 2/5 to –2/5: See Figure 1-65.

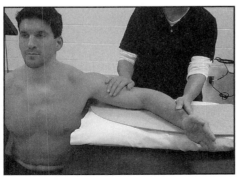

Figure 1-65. The subject flexes the elbow through the maximal available range of motion.

- Grades 1/5 to 0/5: See Figure 1-66.

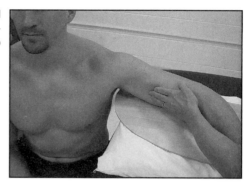

Figure 1-66. The elbow flexors are palpated on the anterior aspect of the arm just proximal to the joint as the subject attempts to flex the elbow.

Substitutions: The subject may extend the shoulder to cause passive flexion to occur or pronate the forearm or flex the wrist during the attempt to flex the elbow.

Points of interest: Rupture of the biceps brachii is often associated with increased age and lifting and is referred to as a "popeye" muscle. Performing a chin-up with the forearm in pronation is more difficult because it places the biceps brachii at a mechanical disadvantage. Of the 3 primary movers, the brachialis is the strongest elbow flexor.

EXTENSION

ACTIVE RANGE OF MOTION

- 145 to 0 degrees (from maximal elbow flexion)

PRIME MOVERS

- Triceps brachii
  - □ Origin:
    - o Long head: Infraglenoid tubercle of the scapula.
    - o Lateral head: Lateral and proximal surface of the upper one half of the humeral shaft above the radial groove.
    - o Medial head: Distal two thirds of the medial and proximal aspects of the humerus below the radial groove.

- Insertion
  - All 3 heads insert onto the olecranon process of the ulna.
- Innervation: Radial nerve (C7 to C8).
- Other actions: Extension of the shoulder.
- Palpation site
  - Long head: Proximal aspect is palpated as it emerges under the posterior deltoid.
  - Lateral head: Distal to the posterior deltoid.
  - Medial head: Distal on the posterior arm on either side of the common triceps tendon.

- Anconeus
  - Origin: Lateral humeral epicondyle.
  - Insertion: Lateral surface of the olecranon process and upper posterior shaft of the ulna.
  - Innervation: Radial nerve (C7 to C8).
  - Other actions: Abduction of the ulna during pronation.
  - Palpation site: Deep to the tendinous sheath of the triceps between the lateral epicondyle and olecranon process of the ulna.

SECONDARY MOVERS
- None

ANTI-GRAVITY
Subject position: Supine on a table with the shoulder flexed to 90 degrees and the elbow in maximal flexion.

Stabilization: The clinician stabilizes the upper arm.

- Grades 5/5 to +3/5: See Figure 1-67.

Figure 1-67. The subject extends the elbow as resistance is applied just proximal to the wrist on the proximal forearm.

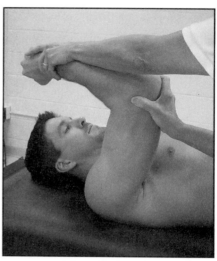

SUBJECT DIRECTIVE: *"Push your arm up toward the ceiling and hold it. Do not let me push it down."*

- Grades 3/5 to +2/5: See Figure 1-68.

Figure 1-68. The subject extends the elbow through the maximal available range of motion without resistance.

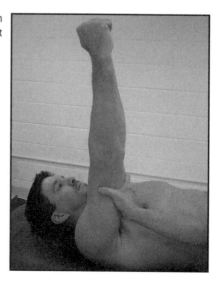

GRAVITY MINIMIZED

Subject position: Sitting with the upper extremity resting on a smooth surface. The shoulder should be in 90 degrees of abduction and internally rotated with the elbow in maximal flexion and forearm in neutral or pronated.

Stabilization: The clinician stabilizes the upper arm.

■ Grades 2/5 to –2/5: See Figure 1-69.

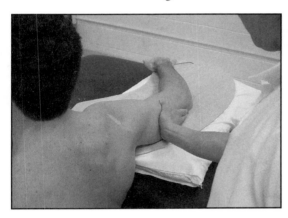

Figure 1-69. The subject extends the elbow through maximal range of motion without resistance.

■ Grades 1/5 to 0/5: See Figure 1-70.

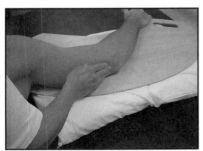

Figure 1-70. The elbow extensors are palpated on the posterior aspect of the arm just proximal to the olecranon.

Substitutions: The subject may attempt to externally rotate or horizontally adduct the shoulder to substitute for a weak triceps brachii muscle.

FOREARM

SUPINATION

ACTIVE RANGE OF MOTION

- 0 to 90 degrees

PRIME MOVERS

- Supinator

    □ Origin: Lateral epicondyle of the humerus, spinator crest of the ulna, and radial collateral and annular ligaments.

    □ Insertion: Lateral surface of the upper third of the radial shaft.

    □ Innervation: Radial nerve (C6 to C7).

    □ Other actions: None.

    □ Palpation site: Distal to the head of the radius on the dorsal aspect of the forearm, under the common extensor muscles off the lateral epicondyle.

SECONDARY MOVERS

- Biceps brachii

ANTI-GRAVITY

Subject position: Sitting with the arm at the subject's side, elbow flexed to 90 degrees, and the forearm in pronation. The fingers should be relaxed.

Stabilization: The clinician stabilizes the upper arm against the trunk.

■ Grades 5/5 to +3/5: See Figure 1-71.

Figure 1-71. Resistance is applied to the wrist just proximal to the joint line into pronation.

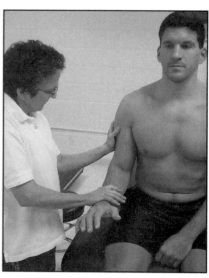

SUBJECT DIRECTIVE: *"Turn your palm up and hold it. Do not let me push it down."*

■ Grades 3/5 to +2/5: See Figure 1-72.

Figure 1-72. The subject supinates the forearm through the available range of motion without resistance.

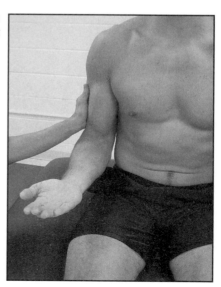

GRAVITY MINIMIZED

Subject position: Sitting with the shoulder in approximately 45 degrees of flexion, the elbow flexed, and the forearm in neutral. The clinician supports the arm at the elbow.

Stabilization: The clinician stabilizes the upper arm against the trunk.

- Grades 2/5 to –2/5: See Figure 1-73.

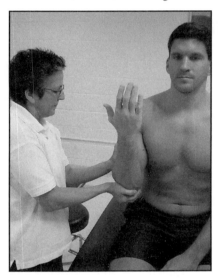

Figure 1-73. The subject supinates the forearm throughout the maximal range of motion.

- Grades 1/5 to 0/5: See Figure 1-74.

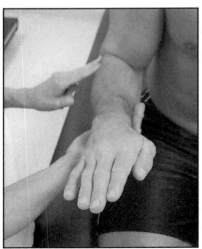

Figure 1-74. The supinator is palpated just distal to the head of the radius on the dorsal aspect of the forearm as the subject attempts to perform the movement.

Substitutions: The subject may try to externally rotate and adduct the shoulder to passively supinate the forearm. The subject may also extend the wrist.

Points of interest: The supinator alone may be active during slow, nonresisted motion. The biceps brachii may be activated to assist if supination with speed or increased resistance is necessary.

PRONATION

ACTIVE RANGE OF MOTION
- 0 to 90 degrees

PRIME MOVERS
- Pronator teres

  □ Origin:

    o Humeral head: Proximal to the medial epicondyle of the humerus.

    o Ulnar head: Medial aspect of the coronoid process of the ulna.

  □ Insertion: Mid-shaft and lateral surface of the radius.

  □ Innervation: Median nerve (C6 to C7).

  □ Other actions: Elbow flexion.

  □ Palpation site: Medial surface of the cubital fossa to the lateral border of the radius.

- Pronator quadratus

  □ Origin: Anterior surface and distal quarter of the ulna.

  □ Insertion: Anterior surface and distal quarter of the radius.

  □ Innervation: Median nerve (C8).

  □ Other actions: None.

  □ Palpation site: Not palpable.

SECONDARY MOVERS
- Flexor carpi radialis

ANTI-GRAVITY
Subject position: Sitting with the arm at the subject's side, elbow flexed to 90 degrees, and the forearm in supination. The fingers should remain relaxed.

Stabilization: The clinician stabilizes the upper arm against the trunk.

■ Grades 5/5 to +3/5: See Figure 1-75.

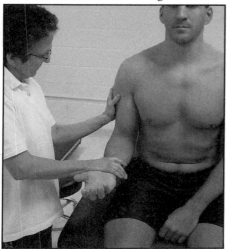

Figure 1-75. Resistance is applied to the wrist just proximal to the joint line into supination.

SUBJECT DIRECTIVE: *"Turn your palm down and hold it. Do not let me push it up."*

■ Grades 3/5 to +2/5: See Figure 1-76.

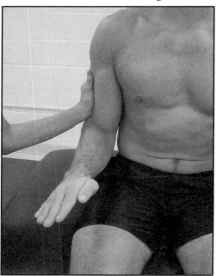

Figure 1-76. The subject pronates the forearm through the maximal range of motion without resistance.

GRAVITY MINIMIZED

Subject position: Sitting with the shoulder in approximately 45 degrees of flexion, the elbow flexed, and forearm in neutral. The clinician supports the arm at the elbow.

Stabilization: The clinician stabilizes the upper arm against the trunk.

- Grades 2/5 to –2/5: See Figure 1-77.

Figure 1-77. The subject pronates the forearm through the maximal available range of motion.

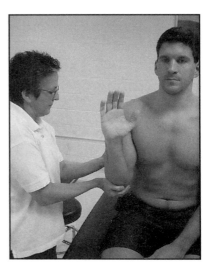

- Grades 1/5 to 0/5: See Figure 1-78.

Figure 1-78. The pronator teres is palpated on the medial surface of the cubital fossa lateral to the radius as the subject attempts to pronate the forearm.

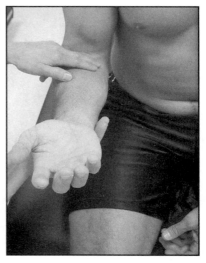

Points of interest: Although both the pronator teres and quadratus are active during pronation of the forearm, the pronator teres becomes more active during explosive activities such as swinging a raquet or pitching a ball. The pronators are functionally associated with shoulder internal rotation because the 2 motions often occur together during activity.

WRIST

FLEXION

ACTIVE RANGE OF MOTION

- 0 to 90 degrees

PRIME MOVERS

- Flexor carpi radialis

  - Origin: Medial epicondyle of the humerus.

  - Insertion: Base of the second metacarpal bone.

  - Innervation: Median nerve (C6 to C7).

  - Other actions: Radially deviates the wrist/hand.

  - Palpation site: Slightly lateral to the midline of the wrist.

- Flexor carpi ulnaris

  - Origin

    - Humeral head: Medial epicondyle from the common flexor tendon.

    - Ulnar head: Medial aspect of the olecranon and proximal border of the ulna.

  - Insertion: Pisiform bone, hamate bone, and base of the fifth metacarpal.

  - Innervation: Ulnar nerve (C7 to C8).

  - Other actions: Ulnarly deviates the wrist/hand.

  - Palpation site: Immediately proximal to the pisiform.

SECONDARY MOVERS

- Palmaris longus
- Flexor digitorum superficialis
- Flexor digitorum profundus
- Abductor pollicis longus
- Flexor pollicis longus

Subject position: Sitting or supine with the forearm supinated and the dorsal surface resting on a tabletop. The wrist should be in neutral with the fingers relaxed.

Stabilization: The clinician stabilizes the forearm against the tabletop.

The flexor carpi radialis and flexor carpi ulnaris may be tested separately by resisting wrist flexion with radial deviation and ulnar deviation, respectively.

- Grades 5/5 to +3/5: See Figure 1-79.

Figure 1-79. Resistance is applied to the palm of the hand into wrist extension.

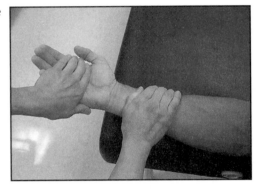

- Grades 3/5 to +2/5: See Figure 1-80.

Figure 1-80. The subject flexes the wrist straight up without deviation through the maximal available range of motion without resistance.

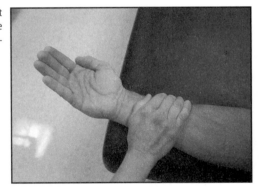

GRAVITY MINIMIZED

Subject position: Sitting or supine with the forearm in neutral and the ulnar border of the hand resting on a tabletop with the wrist in neutral. The fingers should be relaxed.

Stabilization: The clinician stabilizes the forearm against the tabletop.

- Grades 2/5 to –2/5: See Figure 1-81.

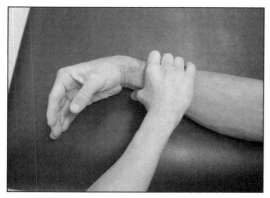

Figure 1-81. The subject flexes the wrist through the maximal range of motion.

- Grades 1/5 to 0/5: See Figure 1-82.

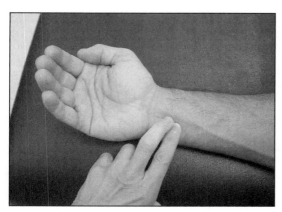

Figure 1-82. The flexor carpi radialis is palpated slightly lateral to the midline of the wrist as the subject attempts to flex and radially deviate the wrist. The flexor carpi ulnaris is palpated immediately proximal to the pisiform as the subject attempts to flex and ulnarly deviate the wrist. (Shown: Palpating the flexor carpi radialis.)

Substitutions: The fingers may flex as the subject attempts to flex the wrist.

EXTENSION

ACTIVE RANGE OF MOTION
- 0 to 70 degrees

PRIME MOVERS
- Extensor carpi radialis longus

  □ Origin: Distal third of the lateral supracondylar ridge of the humerus.

- □ Insertion: Base of the second metacarpal, dorsal surface.

- □ Innervation: Radial nerve (C6 to C7).

- □ Other actions: Radially deviates the wrist/hand.

- □ Palpation site: Radiodorsal aspect of the wrist proximal to the second metacarpal.

- ■ Extensor carpi radialis brevis

  - □ Origin: Lateral epicondyle via the common extensor tendon and radial collateral ligament.

  - □ Insertion: Base of the third metacarpal bone.

  - □ Innervation: Radial nerve (C7 to C8).

  - □ Other actions: Radially deviates the wrist/hand.

  - □ Palpation site: In the depression over the capitate bone as the subject abducts the thumb in the sagittal plane.

- ■ Extensor carpi ulnaris

  - □ Origin: Lateral epicondyle via the common extensor tendon and the posterior aspect of the ulna.

  - □ Insertion: Medial aspect of the base of the fifth metacarpal bone.

  - □ Innervation: Radial nerve (C7 to C8).

  - □ Other actions: Ulnarly deviates the wrist/hand.

  - □ Palpations site: The tendon of the extensor carpi ulnaris is palpated on the ulnar side of the dorsal surface of the wrist just distal to the styloid process of the ulna and proximal to the fifth metacarpal.

SECONDARY MOVERS

- ■ Extensor digitorum

- ■ Extensor digiti minimi

- ■ Extensor indicis

ANTI-GRAVITY

Subject position: Sitting with the forearm pronated and supported on a tabletop. The wrist should be in neutral and the fingers should be relaxed.

Stabilization: The clinician stabilizes the forearm against the tabletop.

The extensor carpi radialis longus, extensor carpi radialis brevis, and extensor carpi ulnaris may be tested separately by resisting wrist extension with radial deviation and ulnar deviation, respectively.

- Grades 5/5 to +3/5: See Figure 1-83.

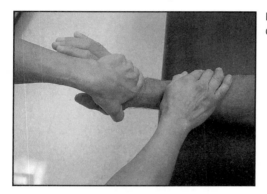

Figure 1-83. Resistance is applied to the dorsum of the hand into wrist flexion.

SUBJECT DIRECTIVE: *"Move the back of your hand up toward the ceiling and hold it. Do not let me push it down."*

- Grades 3/5 to +2/5: See Figure 1-84.

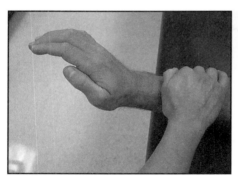

Figure 1-84. The subject extends the wrist straight up without deviation through the maximal available range of motion without resistance.

GRAVITY MINIMIZED

Subject position: Sitting or supine with the forearm in neutral and the ulnar border of the hand resting on a tabletop with the wrist in neutral. The fingers should be relaxed.

- Grades 2/5 to −2/5: See Figure 1-85.

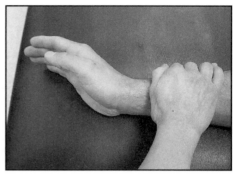

Figure 1-85. The subject extends the wrist through the maximal available range of motion.

- Grades 1/5 to 0/5: See Figure 1-86.

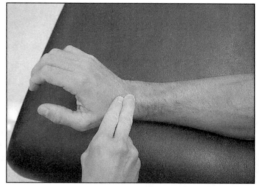

Figure 1-86. The extensor carpi radialis longus is palpated on the dorsum of the wrist in line with the second metacarpal, the extensor carpi radialis is palpated on the dorsum of the wrist in line with the third metacarpal, and the extensor carpi ulnaris is palpated on the dorsum of the wrist proximal to the fifth metacarpal just distal to the ulnar styloid process as the subject attempts to extend and radially or ulnarly deviate the wrist, respectively.
(Shown: Palpating the extensor carpi radialis longus.)

Substitutions: The fingers may extend as the subject attempts to extend the wrist.

FINGERS II TO V

Note: Because gravity is not a significant factor during testing of the fingers/thumb, the format used for grading muscle strength deviates from the standard grading system applied to other muscle groups; half grades are not assigned.

METACARPOPHALANGEAL FLEXION

ACTIVE RANGE OF MOTION
- 0 to 90 degrees

PRIME MOVERS
- Lumbricales

  □ Origin: Originate off of the tendons of the flexor digitorum profundus. Lumbricales #1 and #2: radial sides and plamar surfaces of tendons of digits II and III; #3 is adjacent to sides of digits III and IV; #4 is adjacent to sides of the tendons of digits IV and V.

  □ Insertion: Tendinous expansion of the extensor digitorum, with each muscle running distally to the radial side of the corresponding digit and attaching to the dorsal digital expansion.

  □ Innervation: Lumbricales #1 and #2; median nerve (C8 to T1) and #3 and #4; ulnar nerve (C8 to T1).

  □ Other actions: Extension of the fingers at the proximal interphalangeal (PIP) and distal interphalangeal (DIP) joints.

  □ Palpation site: Not palpable.

SECONDARY MOVERS
- Dorsal/palmar interossei

- Flexor digitorum superficialis

- Flexor digitorum profundus

- Flexor digiti minimi

- Opponens digiti minimi

GRADES 5/5 (NORMAL), 4/5 (GOOD), AND 3/5 (FAIR)

Subject position: Sitting or supine with the forearm in supination and the wrist in neutral. The metacarpophalangeal (MCP) joints should be extended with the PIP and DIP joints flexed.

Stabilization: The clinician stabilizes the metacarpal bones against the tabletop.

- Grades 5/5 to 4/5: See Figure 1-87.

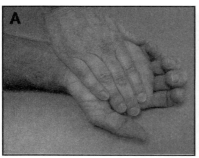 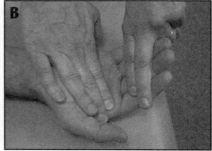

Figure 1-87. Resistance is applied to the palmar surface of the proximal row of the phalanges into metacarpophalangeal extension.

SUBJECT DIRECTIVE: *"Straighten out your fingers as you bend your hand at the knuckles and hold it. Do not let me push your fingers down."*

*The clinician may have to demonstrate the motion first.

- Grade 3/5: See Figure 1-88.

Figure 1-88. The subject flexes the metacarpophalangeal joints while simultaneously extending the proximal and distal interphalangeal joints.

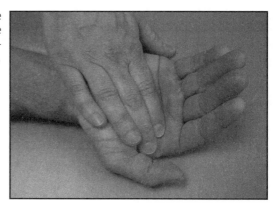

GRADES 2/5 (POOR), 1/5 (TRACE), AND 0/5 (ZERO)

Subject position: Sitting or supine with the forearm and wrist in neutral with the hand resting on the ulnar border. The MCP joints should be maximally extended with the PIP and DIP joints in flexion.

Stabilization: The clinician stabilizes the wrist and hand.

- Grade 2/5: See Figure 1-89.

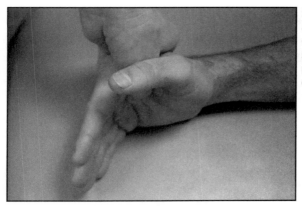

Figure 1-89. The subject attempts to flex the metacarpophalangeal joints while simultaneously extending the proximal interphalangeal and distal interphalangeal joints.

*The lumbricales are too deep to palpate. A grade of 1/5 or trace is given if any movement is observed and 0/5 is assigned in the absence of movement.

Substitutions: The long finger flexors may cause the PIP and DIP joints to flex as the subject attempts to flex the MCP joints.

PIP FLEXION

ACTIVE RANGE OF MOTION

- 0 to 120 degrees

PRIME MOVERS

- Flexor digitorum superficialis

  - Origin: Humero-ulnar head: Medial epicondyle of the humerus and medial aspect of the coronoid process.

  - Radial head: Oblique line of the radius.

  - Insertion: Four tendons insert into each side of the middle phalanx of digits II to V.

  - Innervation: Median nerve (C8 to T1).

  - Other actions: Assists with flexion of the wrist.

  - Palpation site: The tendons are palpated where they cross the palmar surface of each proximal phalanx.

SECONDARY MOVERS

- None

GRADES 5/5 (NORMAL), 4/5 (GOOD), AND 3/5 (FAIR)

Subject position: Sitting or supine with the hand resting on the dorsal side with the wrist in neutral. The tested digit should be slightly flexed at the MCP joint.

Stabilization: All joints of the nontested fingers are held in extension.

- Grades 5/5 to 4/5: See Figure 1-90.

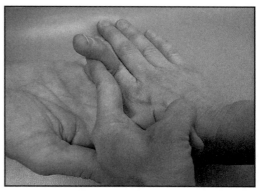

Figure 1-90. Resistance is applied to the palmar surface of the middle phalanx of the tested digit into extension.

SUBJECT DIRECTIVE: *"Bend your finger and hold it. Do not let me straighten it out. Keep all your fingers relaxed."*

- Grade 3/5: See Figure 1-91.

Figure 1-91. The subject flexes the proximal interphalangeal of the tested digit through the maximal available range of motion without resistance.

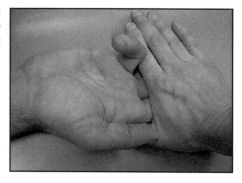

Grades 2/5 (poor), 1/5 (trace), and 0/5 (zero)

Subject position: Sitting or supine with the forearm in neutral and the ulnar border of the hand resting on a tabletop.

Stabilization: The clinician stabilizes the forearm and holds the nontested digits in extension.

- Grade 2/5: See Figure 1-92.

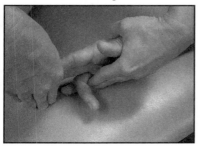

Figure 1-92. The subject flexes the proximal interphalangeal joint of the tested digit through the available range of motion.

- Grades 1/5 to 0/5: See Figure 1-93.

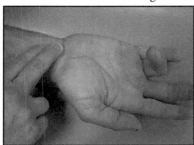

Figure 1-93. The flexor digitorum superficialis is palpated on the palmar aspect of the wrist between the palmaris longus and flexor carpi ulnaris.

Substitutions: The flexor digitorum profundus may cause flexion of the DIP joints as the subject attempts to flex the PIP joint.

DIP FLEXION

ACTIVE RANGE OF MOTION
- 0 to 80 degrees

PRIME MOVERS
- Flexor digitorum profundus

  □ Origin: Anterior and medial surfaces of the proximal three quarters of the ulna.

- Insertion: Four tendons insert into the base of each distal phalanx of digits II to V.

- Ulnar nerve, digits IV and V (C8 to T1).

- Innervation: Median nerve, digits II and III (C8 to T1).

- Other actions: MCP and PIP flexion of fingers II to V. Assists with flexion of the wrist.

- Palpation site: The tendons are palpated where they cross the palmar surface of each middle phalanx of digits II to V.

SECONDARY MOVERS

- None

GRADES 5/5 (NORMAL), 4/5 (GOOD), AND 3/5 (FAIR)

Subject position: Sitting or supine with the hand resting on the dorsal surface with the wrist in neutral. The proximal PIP should be in extension.

Stabilization: The clinician stabilizes the middle phalanx and PIP joint of the tested digit.

- Grades 5/5 to 4/5: See Figure 1-94.

Figure 1-94. Resistance is applied to the palmar surface of the distal phalanx into extension.

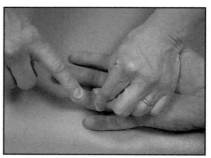

SUBJECT DIRECTIVE: *"Bend the tip of your finger and hold it. Do not let me straighten it out."*

■ Grade 3/5: See Figure 1-95.

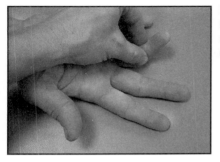

Figure 1-95. The subject flexes the distal interphalangeal of the tested digit through the maximal available range of motion without resistance.

GRADES 2/5 (POOR), 1/5 (TRACE), AND 0/5 (ZERO)

Subject position: Sitting or supine with the forearm in neutral and the ulnar border of the hand resting on a tabletop.

Stabilization: The clinician stabilizes the forearm and holds the middle phalanx of the tested digit in extension.

■ Grade 2/5: See Figure 1-96.

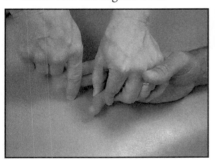

Figure 1-96. The subject flexes the distal interphalangeal joint of the tested digit through the maximal available range of motion.

■ Grades 1/5 to 0/5: See Figure 1-97.

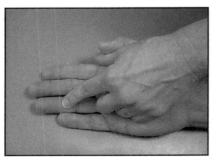

Figure 1-97. The flexor digitorum profundus tendons can be palpated on the palmar surfaces of the middle phalanx of digits II to V.

Substitutions: The wrist must be kept in a neutral position to prevent tenodesis from occurring from wrist extension.

MCP EXTENSION

ACTIVE RANGE OF MOTION

- 90 to 0 degrees (extension from maximal flexion)
- 0 to 30 degrees (hyperextension)

PRIME MOVERS

- Extensor digitorum
  - Origin: Lateral epicondyle of the humerus.
  - Insertion: Via 4 tendons to digits II to V through the extensor hood to the base of the distal phalanx.
  - Innervation: Radial nerve (C7 to C8).
  - Other actions: Extends the PIP joints of fingers II to V. Assists in abduction of fingers I, IV, and V. Assists in the extension and abduction of the wrist.
  - Palpation site: Over the dorsal aspect of the hand as the tendons pass down each finger.
- Extensor indicis
  - Origin: Dorsal surface of the shaft of the ulna below the origin of the extensor pollicis longus.
  - Insertion: Second digit extensor hood via the tendon of the extensor digitorum.
  - Innervation: Radial nerve (C7 to C8).
  - Other actions: Extends the PIP joint of the index finger. Assists in adduction of the index finger and in extension of the wrist.
  - Palpation site: Over the dorsal/ulnar aspect of the second metacarpal, close to the hand.
- Extensor digiti minimi
  - Origin: Lateral epicondyle via the common extensor tendon.

- Insertion: Extensor hood of the fifth finger with the extensor digitorum.

- Innervation: Radial nerve (C7 to C8).

- Other actions: Extends the PIP joint of the little finger and assists with abduction of the little finger. Assists with extension of the wrist.

- Palpation site: Over the dorsal aspect of the fifth metacarpal, close to the head of the ulna.

SECONDARY MOVERS

- None

GRADES 5/5 (NORMAL), 4/5 (GOOD), AND 3/5 (FAIR)

Subject position: Sitting or supine with the forearm in pronation and the wrist in neutral with the palmar aspect of the hand resting on a tabletop and the MCP joints flexed to 90 degrees off the edge of the table.

Stabilization: The clinician stabilizes the hand and wrist.

- Grades 5/5 to 4/5: See Figure 1-98.

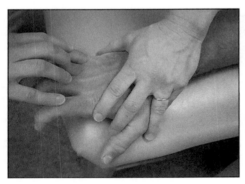

Figure 1-98. Resistance is applied to the distal end of the proximal phalanx (dorsally) as the subject extends the MCP joints with the PIP joints in flexion.

To test the extensor indicis and extensor digiti minimi, the subject extends the MCP joint of the second digit and fifth digit, respectively.

SUBJECT DIRECTIVE: *"Bend your knuckles up and hold it. Do not let me push them down."*

The clinician may have to demonstrate the motion first.

- Grade 3/5: See Figure 1-99.

Figure 1-99. The subject extends the tested metacarpophalangeal joints through the maximal range of motion without resistance.

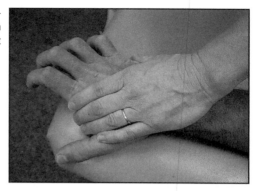

GRADES 2/5 (POOR), 1/5 (TRACE), AND 0/5 (ZERO)

Subject position: Sitting or supine with the forearm and wrist in neutral with the hand resting on the ulnar border on a tabletop.

- Grade 2/5: See Figure 1-100.

Figure 1-100. The subject extends the metacarpophalangeal joint of the tested digits through the maximal range of motion.

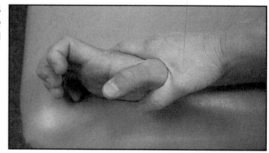

- Grades 1/5 to 0/5: See Figure 1-101.

Figure 1-101. The tendons of the extensor digitorum, extensor indicis, and extensor digiti minimi are readily palpable on the dorsal surface of the hand as the subject attempts to extend the corresponding metacarpophalangeal joints.
(Shown: palpating the tendons of the extensor digitorum.)

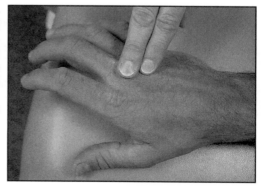

Substitution: Flexion of the wrist may cause interphalangeal (IP) extension via tenodesis. Substitution by the lumbricals may also cause extension of the IP joints.

FINGER ABDUCTION

ACTIVE RANGE OF MOTION
- 0 to 20 degrees

PRIME MOVERS
- Dorsal interossei

  □ Origin: Between each metacarpal bone on adjacent sides.

  □ Insertion:

    o First/second: Radial side of the extensor expansion of the second and third digits.

    o Third/fourth: Ulnar side of the extensor expansion of the third and fourth digits.

  □ Innervation: Ulnar nerve (C8 to T1).

  □ Other actions: Assists the lumbricals in MCP flexion and PIP/DIP extension of fingers II to V.

  □ Palpation site: First dorsal interossei-radial side of the second meta-carpal; second dorsal interossei-radial side of the proximal phalanx of the third digit; third dorsal interossei-ulnar side of the proximal phalanx of the third digit; fourth dorsal interossei-ulnar side of the proximal phalanx of the fourth digit.

- Abductor digiti minimi

  □ Origin: Pisiform bone and tendon of the flexor carpi ulnaris muscle.

  □ Insertion: Base of the proximal phalanx of the fifth digit (ulnar side) and dorsal expansion of the extensor digiti minimi.

  □ Innervation: Ulnar side (C8 to T1).

  □ Other actions: Assists with extension of the wrist.

  □ Palpation site: Along the ulnar border of the fifth metacarpal.

SECONDARY MOVERS

- Extensor digitorum

- Extensor digiti minimi

GRADES 5/5 (NORMAL), 4/5 (GOOD), AND 3/5 (FAIR)

Subject position: Sitting or supine with the forearm pronated, wrist in neutral, and the palmar aspect of the hand resting on the tabletop. The fingers should be in extension.

Stabilization: The clinician stabilizes the hand and nontested fingers.

- Grades 5/5 to 4/5: See Figure 1-102.

Figure 1-102. Resistance is applied to the radial side of one finger and ulnar side of the adjacent finger on the distal end of the proximal phalanx into finger adduction.

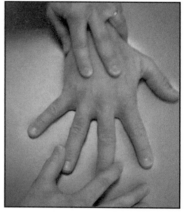

SUBJECT DIRECTIVE: *"Spread your fingers apart and hold it. Do not let me push them together."*

- Grade 3/5: See Figure 1-103.

Figure 1-103. The subject abducts the tested fingers through the maximal range of motion without resistance.

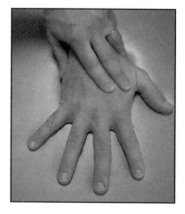

Because the third digit has 2 dorsal interossei, it is important that it is tested as it moves away from the midline in both directions (ulnarly and radially).

GRADES 2/5 (POOR), 1/5 (TRACE), AND 0/5 (ZERO)

Subject position: Sitting or supine with the forearm pronated, wrist in neutral, and the palmar aspect of the hand resting on the table. The fingers should be in extension.

Stabilization: The clinician stabilizes the hand (and nontested fingers when testing fingers individually.)

- Grade 2/5: See Figure 1-104.

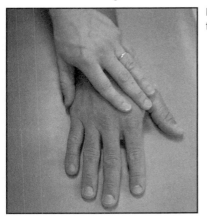

Figure 1-104. The subject is able to abduct the tested fingers through partial range of motion.

- Grades 1/5 to 0/5: See Figure 1-105.

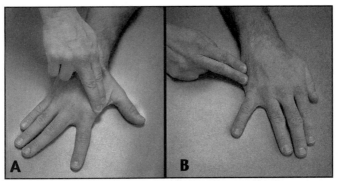

Figure 1-105. The dorsal interossei are palpated for the corresponding digit as the subject attempts to abduct the finger. (A) Palpating the first dorsal interossei and (B) palpating the abductor digiti minimi.

The most readily palpable dorsal interossei muscle is the first, which is located at the base of the proximal phalanx. The abductor digiti minimi is palpated on the ulnar border of the hand as the subject abducts the fifth digit.

Substitutions: The subject may try to extend the MCP joints as he or she attempts to abduct the fingers.

FINGER ADDUCTION

ACTIVE RANGE OF MOTION

- 0 to 20 degrees

PRIME MOVERS

- Palmar interossei

  □ Origin

    o First: Length of the ulnar side of the second metacarpal.

    o Second: Length of the radial side of the fourth metacarpal.

    o Third: Length of the radial side of the fifth metacarpal.

  □ Insertion

    o First: Proximal phalanx, ulnar side of the second digit.

    o Second: Proximal phalanx, radial side of the fourth digit.

    o Third: Proximal phalanx, radial side of the fifth digit.

  □ Innervation: Ulnar nerve (C8 to T1),

  □ Other actions: Assists the lumbricals in MCP flexion and PIP/DIP extension of fingers II to V.

  □ Palpation site: First palmar interossei-ulnar side of the proximal phalanx of the second digit; second palmar interossei-radial side of the proximal phalanx of the fourth digit; third palmar interossei-radial side of the proximal phalanx of the fifth digit.

SECONDARY MOVERS

- Extensor indicis

GRADES 5/5 (NORMAL), 4/5 (GOOD), AND 3/5 (FAIR)

Subject position: Sitting or supine with the forearm pronated, wrist in neutral, and the palmar aspect of the hand resting on a tabletop. The fingers should be in extension.

Stabilization: The clinician stabilizes the hand and nontested fingers.

- Grades 5/5 to 4/5: See Figure 1-106.

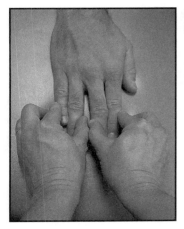

Figure 1-106. Resistance is applied to the middle phalanx of each of the 2 adjoining fingers, "pulling" them into abduction.

SUBJECT DIRECTIVE: *"Keep your fingers together and do not let me pull them apart."*

*The third digit has no palmar interosseus and is not tested in adduction.

- Grade 3/5: See Figure 1-107.

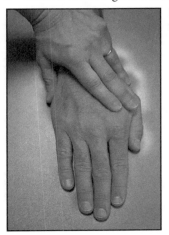

Figure 1-107. The subject is able to adduct the fingers toward the middle finger but is unable to hold them against resistance.

GRADES 2/5 (POOR), 1/5 (TRACE), AND 0/5 (ZERO)

Subject position: Sitting or supine with the forearm pronated, wrist in neutral, and the palmar aspect of the hand resting on a tabletop. The fingers should be in extension and abducted.

Stabilization: The clinician stabilizes the hand and nontested fingers.

- Grade 2/5: See Figure 1-108.

Figure 1-108. The subject is able to adduct the tested finger through partial range of motion.

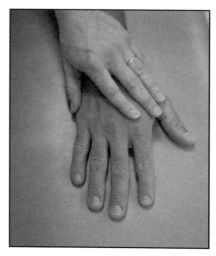

- Grades 1/5 to 0/5: See Figure 1-109.

Figure 1-109. The palmar interossei are difficult to palpate, but the clinician might be able to detect a slight contraction by placing a finger against the side of the finger to be tested.

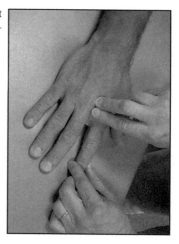

Substitutions: The subject might flex the fingers while attempting to move them into adduction.

THUMB

MCP FLEXION

ACTIVE RANGE OF MOTION

- 0 to 50 degrees (MCP flexion)

PRIME MOVERS

- Flexor pollicis brevis

  □ Origin: Distal ridge of the trapezium, the trapezoid, capitate, and flexor retinaculum.

  □ Insertion: Base of the proximal phalanx of the thumb on the radial side.

  □ Innervation: Median nerve (C8 to T1).

  □ Other actions: None.

  □ Palpation site: The ulnar side of the first metacarpal.

SECONDARY MOVERS

- None

GRADES 5/5 (NORMAL), 4/5 (GOOD), AND 3/5 (FAIR)

Subject position: Sitting or supine with the forearm in supination, the wrist in neutral, and the hand resting on the dorsal surface on a tabletop. The thumb is in an adducted position.

Stabilization: The clinician stabilizes the first metacarpal.

- Grades 5/5 to 4/5: See Figure 1-110.

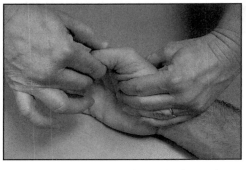

Figure 1-110. Resistance is applied to the proximal phalanx into extension.

SUBJECT DIRECTIVE: *"Bend the base of your thumb and hold it. Do not let me straighten it out."*

*For a grade of 3/5, the subject flexes the MCP through the maximal range of motion with slight resistance.

GRADES 2/5 (POOR), 1/5 (TRACE), AND 0/5 (ZERO)

- Grade 2/5: See Figure 1-111.

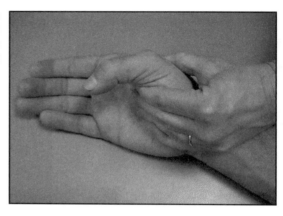

Figure 1-111. The subject flexes both the metacarpophalangeal joint of the thumb through maximal range of motion without resistance.

- Grades 1/5 to 0/5: See Figure 1-112.

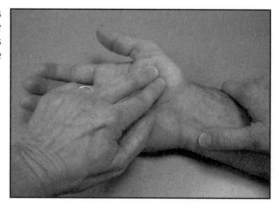

Figure 1-112. The flexor pollicis brevis is palpated on the ulnar side of the first metacarpal as the subject attempts to flex the metacarpophalangeal joint.

Substitutions: The flexor pollicis longus may be activated to flex the MCP joint. The DIP of the thumb should remain in extension during testing of MCP flexion to avoid this substitution.

IP FLEXION

ACTIVE RANGE OF MOTION

- 0 to 90 degrees

PRIME MOVERS

- Flexor pollicis longus

    □ Origin: Anterior surface of the middle half of the shaft of the radius and coronoid process of the ulna.

    □ Insertion: Base of the distal phalanx of the thumb.

    □ Innervation: Median nerve (C8 to T1).

    □ Other actions: None.

    □ Palpation site: Palpate where the tendon crosses the palmar surface of the proximal phalanx of the thumb.

SECONDARY MOVERS

- None

GRADES 5/5 (NORMAL), 4/5 (GOOD), AND 3/5 (FAIR)

Subject position: Sitting or supine with the forearm in supination, the wrist in neutral, and the hand resting on the dorsal surface on a tabletop. The thumb is in an adducted position.

Stabilization: The clinician stabilizes the proximal phalanx.

- Grades 5/5 to 4/5: See Figure 1-113.

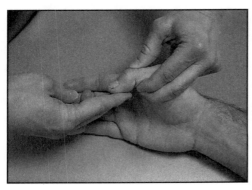

Figure 1-113. Resistance is applied to the distal phalanx into extension.

SUBJECT DIRECTIVE: *"Bend the tip of your thumb and hold it. Do not let me straighten it out."*

For a grade of 3/5, the subject flexes the IP joint through the maximal range of motion with slight resistance.

GRADES 2/5 (POOR), 1/5 (TRACE), AND 0/5 (ZERO)

- Grade 2/5: See Figure 1-114.

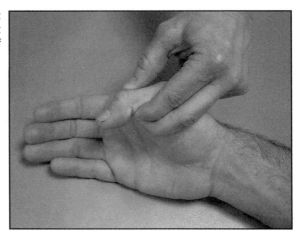

Figure 1-114. The subject flexes the interphalangeal joint through the maximal range of motion without resistance.

- Grades 1/5 to 0/5: See Figure 1-115.

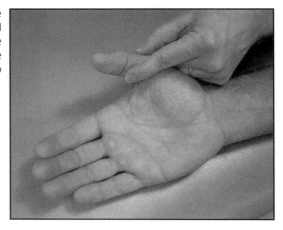

Figure 1-115. The tendon of the flexor pollicis longus is palpated where it crosses the palmar surface of the proximal phalanx of the thumb as the subject attempts to flex the interphalangeal joint.

MCP EXTENSION

ACTIVE RANGE OF MOTION

- 50 to 0 degrees (MCP extension)

PRIME MOVERS

- Extensor pollicis brevis

  □ Origin: Dorsal surface of the distal radius.

  □ Insertion: Base of the first proximal phalanx of the thumb.

  □ Innervation: Radial nerve (C7 to C8).

  □ Other actions: Assists with wrist radial deviation.

  □ Palpation site: Palpate the tendon of the extensor pollicis brevis as it crosses the lateral aspect of the base of the first MCP.

SECONDARY MOVERS

- None

Grades 5/5 (normal), 4/5 (good), and 3/5 (fair)

Subject position: Sitting or supine with the forearm and wrist in neutral and the hand resting on the ulnar border on a tabletop.

Stabilization: The clinician stabilizes the first metacarpal.

- Grades 5/5 to 4/5: See Figure 1-116.

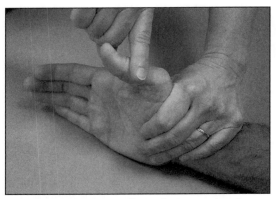

Figure 1-116. Resistance is applied to the dorsal surface of the proximal phalanx.

SUBJECT DIRECTIVE: *"Straighten your thumb out and hold it. Do not let me push it down."*

For a grade of 3/5, the subject extends the MCP joint through the maximal range of motion with slight resistance.

GRADES 2/5 (POOR), 1/5 (TRACE), AND 0/5 (ZERO)

Subject position: Sitting or supine with the forearm and wrist in neutral and the hand resting on the ulnar border on a tabletop.

Stabilization: The clinician stabilizes the first metacarpal.

- Grade 2/5: See Figure 1-117.

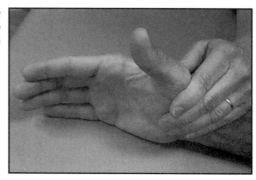

Figure 1-117. The subject extends the metacarpophalangeal joint of the thumb through maximal range of motion without resistance.

- Grades 1/5 to 0/5: See Figure 1-118.

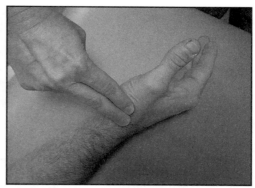

Figure 1-118. The extensor pollicis brevis is palpated at the base of the first metacarpal between the tendons of the abductor pollicis and extensor pollicis longus as the subject attempts to extend the first metacarpophalangeal joint. (Shown: Palpating the extensor pollicis brevis.)

Substitutions: If the extensor pollicis longus comes into play while the subject is attempting to extend the first MCP joint, the clinician may observe the IP joint of the thumb extend as the carpometacarpal (CMC) joint adducts.

IP EXTENSION

ACTIVE RANGE OF MOTION

- 90 to 0 degrees

PRIME MOVERS

- Extensor pollicis longus

  - □ Origin: Lateral aspect of the middle third of the dorsal surface of the ulna.

  - □ Insertion: Base of the first proximal phalanx of the thumb.

  - □ Innervation: Radial nerve (C7 to C8).

  - □ Other actions: Assists with radial deviation.

  - □ Palpation site: Palpate the tendon of the extensor pollicis longus as it crosses the dorsal aspect at the base of the first MCP.

SECONDARY MOVERS

- None

Grades 5/5 (normal), 4/5 (good), and 3/5 (fair)

Subject position: Sitting or supine with the forearm and wrist in neutral and the hand resting on the ulnar border on a tabletop.

Stabilization: The clinician stabilizes the proximal phalanx.

- Grades 5/5 to 4/5: See Figure 1-119.

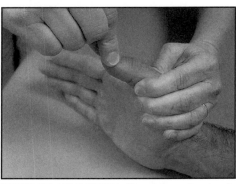

Figure 1-119. Resistance is applied to the dorsal surface of the distal phalanx.

SUBJECT DIRECTIVE: *"Straighten the tip of your thumb out and hold it. Do not let me bend it down."*

*For a grade of 3/5, the subject extends the IP joint through the maximal range of motion with slight resistance.

Grades 2/5 (poor), 1/5 (trace), and 0/5 (zero)

Subject position: Sitting or supine with the forearm and wrist in neutral and the hand resting on the ulnar border on a tabletop.

Stabilization: The clinician stabilizes the proximal phalanx and metacarpal.

- Grade 2/5: See Figure 1-120.

Figure 1-120. The subject extends the interphalangeal joint through the range of motion without resistance.

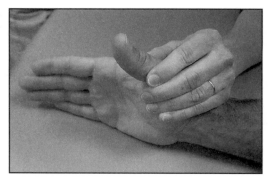

- Grades 1/5 to 0/5: See Figure 1-121.

Figure 1-121. The extensor pollicis longus is palpated on the ulnar aspect of the "anatomical snuff box" on the dorsal surface at the base of the first metacarpal as the subject attempts to extend the first interphalangeal joint.

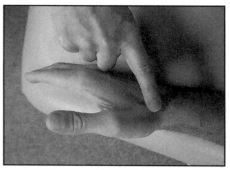

Substitutions: The muscles of the thenar eminence may be activated to flex the CMC joint, resulting in IP joint extension via extensor tenodesis.

THUMB ABDUCTION

ACTIVE RANGE OF MOTION

- 0 to 60 degrees

PRIME MOVERS

- Abductor pollicis brevis

    □ Origin: Flexor retinaculum, scaphoid, and trapezium tubercles.

    □ Insertion: Base of the first proximal phalanx, radial aspect.

    □ Innervation: Median nerve (C8 to T1).

- ☐ Other actions: None.
- ☐ Palpation site: Along the anterior surface of the shaft of the first metacarpal.

■ Abductor pollicis longus

- ☐ Origin: Lateral aspect of the dorsal surface of the shaft of the ulna.
- ☐ Insertion: Base of the first metacarpal, radial aspect.
- ☐ Innervation: Radial nerve (C7 to C8).
- ☐ Other actions: Assists with wrist radial deviation.
- ☐ Palpation site: The most anterior of the 3 tendons at the base of the CMC joint; palpate immediately proximal to the CMC joint.

SECONDARY MOVERS

- ■ Palmaris longus
- ■ Extensor pollicis brevis
- ■ Opponens pollicis

GRADES 5/5 (NORMAL), 4/5 (GOOD), AND 3/5 (FAIR)

Subject position: Sitting or supine with the forearm supinated and wrist in neutral with the hand resting on the dorsal surface; thumb relaxed into adduction. The MCP and IP joints should be flexed when testing the abductor pollicis longus to decrease thumb extension.

Stabilization: The clinician stabilizes the palm of the hand and wrist.

- ■ Grades 5/5 to 4/5: See Figures 1-122.

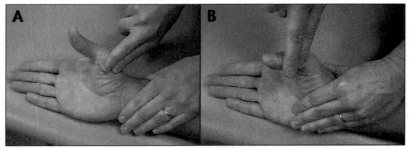

Figures 1-122. (A) Resistance is applied to the distal end of the first metacarpal into adduction to test the abductor pollicis longus and (B) the proximal phalanx for the abductor pollicis brevis.

SUBJECT DIRECTIVE: *"Move your thumb away from your palm toward the ceiling and hold it. Do not let me push it down."*

- Grade 3/5: See Figure 1-123.

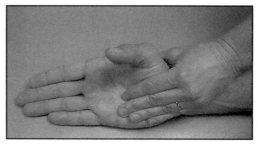

Figure 1-123. The subject abducts the thumb through the maximal range of motion without resistance.

GRADES 2/5 (POOR), 1/5 (TRACE), AND 0/5 (ZERO)

Subject position: Sitting or supine with the forearm in neutral and wrist in neutral with the hand resting on the ulnar border, thumb relaxed into adduction.

Stabilization: The clinician stabilizes the palm of the hand and wrist.

- Grade 2/5: See Figure 1-124.

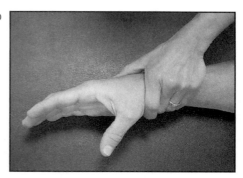

Figure 1-124. The subject abducts the thumb through maximal range of motion.

- Grades 1/5 to 0/5: See Figure 1-125.

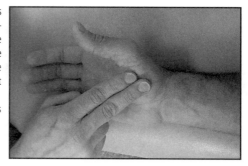

Figure 1-125. The abductor pollicis brevis is palpated in the center of the thenar eminence, medial to the opponens, and the abductor pollicis longus is palpated at the base of the first metacarpal on the radial side of the extensor pollicis brevis as the subject attempts to abduct the thumb.
(Shown: Palpating the abductor pollicis brevis.)

Substitution: If the thumb deviates toward the dorsal surface of the forearm, the extensor pollicis brevis is being called in to substitute for the abductor pollicis longus.

The thumb will deviate radially if the abductor pollicis longus is stronger than the brevis and ulnarly if the abductor pollicis brevis is stronger than the longus.

THUMB ADDUCTION

ACTIVE RANGE OF MOTION

- 60 to 0 degrees

PRIME MOVERS

- Adductor pollicis

    □ Origin: Capitate bone and bases of the second and third metacarpal bones and palmar surface of the distal two thirds of the third metacarpal bone.

    □ Insertion: Ulnar aspect of the base of the proximal phalanx of the thumb.

    □ Innervation: Ulnar nerve (C8 to T1).

    □ Other actions: None.

    □ Palpation site: Deep in the first web space between the first dorsal interossei and the first metacarpal bone.

SECONDARY MOVERS

- First dorsal interosseus

GRADES 5/5 (NORMAL), 4/5 (GOOD), AND 3/5 (FAIR)

Subject position: Sitting or supine with the forearm in pronation and the hand hanging over the edge of a table, supported by the clinician's hand. The wrist is in neutral with the thumb positioned loosely in abduction.

Stabilization: The clinician stabilizes the palm of the hand.

- Grades 5/5 to 4/5: See Figure 1-126.

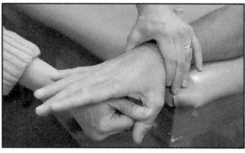

Figure 1-126. Resistance is applied on the medial aspect of the proximal phalanx of the thumb into abduction.

SUBJECT DIRECTIVE: *"Move your thumb in toward your index finger and hold it. Do not let me move it out."*

- Grade 3/5: See Figure 1-127.

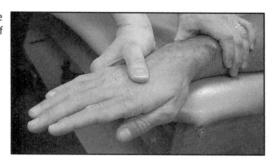

Figure 1-127. The subject adducts the thumb through the maximal range of motion without resistance.

GRADES 2/5 (POOR), 1/5 (GOOD), AND 0/5 (ZERO)

Subject position: Sitting or supine with the forearm and wrist in neutral with the ulnar border of the hand resting on the tabletop with the thumb in abduction.

Stabilization: The clinician stabilizes the wrist and hand on the tabletop.

- Grade 2/5: See Figure 1-128.

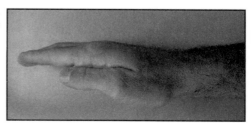

Figure 1-128. The subject adducts the thumb through the maximal range of motion.

- Grades 1/5 to 0/5: See Figure 1-129.

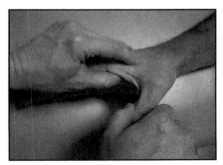

Figure 1-129. The adductor pollicis is palpated on the palmar aspect of the first web space between the first dorsal interosseus and the first metacarpal bone by grasping the web space between the index finger and thumb.

Substitutions: The CMC joint will extend if the extensor pollicis longus is activated while the subject attempts to adduct the thumb and flexor pollicis brevis and longus may flex the thumb as the thumb is adducted.

THUMB OPPOSITION

ACTIVE RANGE OF MOTION

- Variable; "normal" range of motion allows for complete motion until the tips of the thumb and fifth digit meet from an open palm position.

PRIMARY MOVERS

- Opponens pollicis

  □ Origin: Tuberosity of the trapezium and flexor retinaculum.

  □ Insertion: Entire lateral aspect of the shaft of the first metacarpal bone.

  □ Innervation: Median nerve (C8 to T1).

  □ Other actions: None.

  □ Palpation site: Deep to the abductor pollicis brevis along the lateral shaft of the first metacarpal.

- Opponens digiti minimi

  □ Origin: Hook of the hamate and flexor retinaculum.

  □ Insertion: The entire ulnar margin of the shaft of the fifth metacarpal.

  □ Innervation: (C8 to T1).

- □ Other actions: None.

- □ Palpation site: Along the shaft of the fifth metacarpal deep to the abductor digiti minimi.

SECONDARY MOVERS

- ■ Abductor pollicis brevis

- ■ Flexor pollicis brevis

GRADES 5/5 (NORMAL), 4/5 (GOOD), AND 3/5 (FAIR)

Subject position: Sitting or supine with the forearm in supination with the wrist in neutral, thumb adducted, and the MCP and IP joints in flexion.

Stabilization: The clinician stabilizes the hand and wrist against the table-top if necessary.

- ■ Grades 5/5 to 4/5: See Figure 1-130.

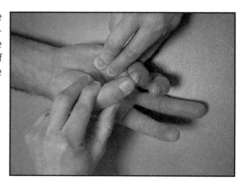

Figure 1-130. Resistance is applied at the head of the first metacarpal into lateral rotation, extension, and adduction to test the opponens pollicis and the palmar surface of the fifth metacarpal (trying to "flatten" the palm) for the opponens digiti minimi.

SUBJECT DIRECTIVE: *"Put the pads of your thumb and little finger together so they meet in the shape of an 'O' and do not let me pull them apart."*

- ■ Grade 3/5: See Figure 1-131.

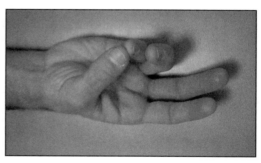

Figure 1-131. The subject is able to move the thumb away from the palm and rotate it so that the pad of the thumb touches the pad of the fifth digit.

GRADES 2/5 (POOR), 1/5 (TRACE), AND 0/5 (ZERO)

Subject position: Sitting or supine with the forearm in supination with the wrist in neutral, thumb adducted and the MCP and IP joints in flexion.

Stabilization: The clinician stabilizes the hand and wrist against the table-top if necessary. Grade 2/5: Not pictured. The two opponens muscles move through the range of motion, but are evaluated individually.

- Grades 1/5 to 0/5: See Figure 1-132.

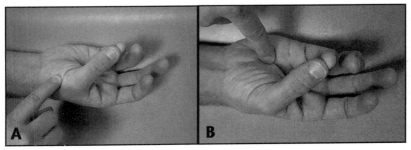

Figure 1-132. (A) The opponens pollicis may be palpated along the radial aspect of the first metacarpal, lateral to the abductor pollicis brevis. (B) The opponens digiti minimi may be palpated on the radial aspect of the fifth metacarpal as the subject attempts to oppose the thumb.

Substitutions: If the thumb moves parallel to the surface of the palm toward the little finger and touches the tips, not the pads of the fingers, the flexor pollicis longus and brevis have been activated. This is not considered opposition of the thumb.

SECTION II

Trunk / Lower Extremities

Van Ost, L.
*Cram Session in Manual Muscle Testing:
A Handbook for Students & Clinicians* (pp. 99-178)
© 2012 SLACK Incorporated

TRUNK

FLEXION

PRIME MOVERS

- Rectus abdominus

  - □ Origin: Pubic crest and symphysis.

  - □ Insertion: Costal cartilage of ribs 5 to 7 and the xiphoid process of the sternum.

  - □ Innervation: Ventral primary rami (T5 to L1).

  - □ Other actions: None.

  - □ Palpation sites: Upper rectus: both sides of the midline between the umbilicus and xiphoid process. Lower rectus: both sides of the midline between the umbilicus and symphysis pubis.

- External oblique

  - □ Origin: Lateral surface of ribs 5 to 12.

  - □ Insertion: Linea alba, inguinal ligament, anterior superior iliac spine, pubic tubercle, and anterior half of the iliac crest.

  - □ Innervation: Ventral primary rami (T5 to L1).

  - □ Other actions: Trunk rotation.

  - □ Palpation site: Opposite side of direction of rotation just below the ribs and lateral to the rectus abdominus.

- Internal oblique

  - □ Origin: Inguinal ligament, iliac crest, and the thoracolumbar fascia.

  - □ Insertion: Pubic crest, linea alba, and ribs 10 to 12.

  - □ Innervation: Ventral primary rami (T7 to L1).

  - □ Other actions: Trunk rotation.

  - □ Palpation site: Just medial to the anterior superior iliac spine along the lateral aspect of the abdomen.

SECONDARY MOVERS

- Psoas major
- Psoas minor

ANTI-GRAVITY

■ Upper rectus abdominus

Subject position: Supine on a table with both lower extremities in extension.

Stabilization: No stabilization of the pelvis is provided if the hip flexors are strong. If weak hip flexors are noted, the clinician stabilizes the pelvis against the table.

■ Grade 5/5: See Figure 2-1.

Figure 2-1. With the hands clasped behind the head, the subject moves through the range of motion until the inferior angles of the scapulae are off the table. The arms create the resistance.

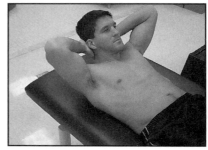

SUBJECT DIRECTIVE: *"Curl your head, shoulders, and torso up until your shoulder blades are off the table."*

■ Grades 4/5 and 3/5: See Figures 2-2 and 2-3.

Figure 2-2. With the arms crossed over the chest, the subject moves through the range of motion until the inferior angles of the scapulae are off the table for a grade of 4/5.

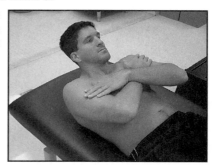

Figure 2-3. With the arms fully outstretched over the trunk, the subject completes the range of motion until the inferior angles of the scapulae are off the table for a grade of 3/5.

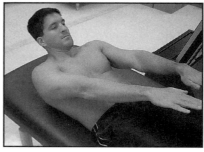

Substitutions: The subject may rise up rapidly to use momentum to lift the trunk or use his arms to push off the tabletop. If the subject inhales deeply, it may cause depression of the lower thorax. The umbilicus may deviate to the stronger side.

GRAVITY MINIMIZED

- Upper rectus abdominis

Subject position: Supine on a table with the knees flexed.

Stabilization: The clinician stabilizes the subject's pelvis against the table.

- Grade 2/5: See Figure 2-4.

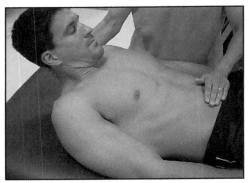

Figure 2-4. The subject is able to raise his head against gravity.

- Grade 1/5: See Figure 2-5.

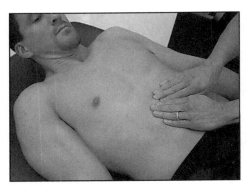

Figure 2-5. If there is no depression of the rib cage but there is visable muscle activity noted, contraction of the upper rectus abdominis is palpated on both sides of the midline between the umbilicus and xiphoid process.

ANTI-GRAVITY

- Lower rectus abdominus

Subject position: Supine on a table with both knees flexed.

Stabilization: The weight of the pelvis and lower extremities provide the necessary stabilization. See Figure 2-6.

Figure 2-6. The subject is able to bring both knees toward the chest and lift the sacrum through the maximal range of motion 10 times for a grade of 5/5 and 4 to 6 times for a grade of 4/5. A grade of 3/5 is assigned if the subject can only complete the motion once.

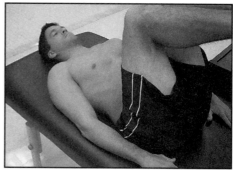

SUBJECT DIRECTIVE: *"Lift both your knees toward your chest and lift your buttocks off the table."*

Substitutions: The subject may use the arms to push up or use momentum to lift up the sacrum. The umbilicus may deviate to the stronger side.

GRAVITY MINIMIZED

- Lower rectus abdominis

Subject position: Supine on a table with the knees flexed.

Stabilization: The weight of the trunk and lower extremities stabilizes the subject's pelvis against the table. See Figures 2-7 and 2-8.

Figure 2-7. Subject is able to perform a pelvic tilt for a grade of 2/5.

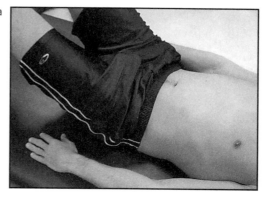

Points of interest: The rectus abdominis and internal and external obliques act together to stabilize the pelvis and contribute to proper postural alignment. Weakness of the abdominal obliques may decrease respiratory efficiency and reduce support of the abdominal viscera.

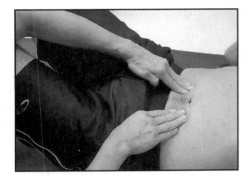

Figure 2-8. Contraction of the lower rectus abdominis is palpated on both sides of the midline between the umbilicus and symphysis pubis for a grade of 1/5.

ROTATION

PRIME MOVERS

- External oblique

  □ Origin: Lateral surface of ribs 5 to 12.

  □ Insertion: Linea alba, inguinal ligament, anterior superior iliac spine, pubic tubercle, and anterior half of the iliac crest.

  □ Innervation: Ventral primary rami of T7 to L1.

  □ Other actions: Trunk flexion.

  □ Palpation site: Below the ribs and costal cartilages of the lowest ribs in the midclavicular line.

- Internal oblique

  □ Origin: Inguinal ligament, iliac crest, and the thoracolumbar fascia.

  □ Insertion: Pubic crest, linea alba, and ribs 10 to 12.

  □ Innervation: Ventral primary rami of T7 to L1.

  □ Other actions: Trunk flexion.

  □ Palpation site: Immediately medial to the anterior superior iliac spine along the midclavicular line.

SECONDARY MOVERS

- None

ANTI-GRAVITY

Subject position: Supine on a table with the lower extremities extended.

Stabilization: The clinician stabilizes the pelvis against the table.

The scapula corresponding to the external oblique must clear the table for a grade of 5/5. See Figure 2-9.

Figure 2-9. With the hands clasped behind the head, the subject flexes the trunk and rotates to one side first and then to the opposite side.

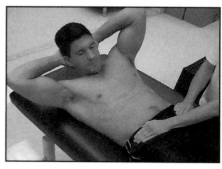

SUBJECT DIRECTIVE: *"Lift your head and shoulders off the table and turn to your left elbow toward your right knee."*

- Grades 4/5 and 3/5: See Figures 2-10 and 2-11.

*Instruct the subject to turn the right elbow toward the left knee to test the opposite side/musculature. When moving the right elbow toward the left knee, the right external and left internal obliques are tested.

Figure 2-10. The subject completes the movement with the hands crossed over the chest for a grade of 4/5.

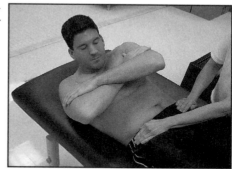

Figure 2-11. The subject completes the movement with the arms outstretched in front of the body for a grade of 3/5.

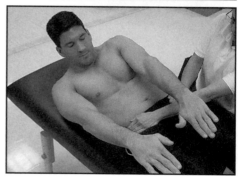

Substitutions: The pectoralis major may cause the shoulders to shrug or slightly lift the shoulder off the table.

GRAVITY MINIMIZED

Subject position: Supine on the table with the lower extremities extended.

Stabilization: The clinician stabilizes the pelvis against the table. See Figure 2-12.

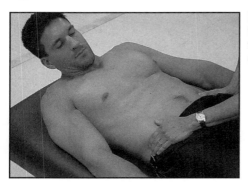

Figure 2-12. The subject is able to initiate the elevation of the opposite scapula with the upper extremities by the sides for a grade of +2/5.

- Grades 1/5 to 0/5: See Figure 2-13.

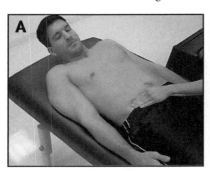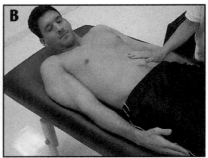

Figures 2-13. (A) The internal obliques are palpated on the side toward which the patient turns just medial to the ASIS on the lateral aspect of the abdomen. (B) The external obliques are palpated on the side away from the direction of turning just below the ribs and lateral to the rectus abdominus.

*The umbilicus will move toward the strongest quadrant when there is unequal strength in the opposing obliques.

Note: The direction of the muscle fibers of the internal obliques can be mimicked by crossing the arms over the abdomen and placing the fingertips on each anterior superior iliac spine. The fingers will parallel the muscle fibers (up and in). The direction of the muscle fibers of the external obliques can be mimicked by positioning the hands into the pants pockets (down and in).

EXTENSION

PRIME MOVERS

Note: Palpation sites are not listed as the individual muscles cannot be isolated.

- Iliocostalis thoracis

  □ Origin: Angles of ribs 7 to 12.

  □ Insertion: Angles of ribs 6 to 1 and the transverse process of C7.

  □ Innervation: Dorsal primary rami of the thoracic spinal nerves.

  □ Other actions: Trunk lateral flexion.

- Longissimus thoracis

  □ Origin: Lumbar transverse processes (L1 to L5) and thoracolumbar fascia.

  □ Insertion: Transverse processes of T1 to T12 and ribs 2 to 12 between the angles and tubercles.

  □ Innervation: Dorsal primary rami of the thoracic spinal nerves.

  □ Other actions: None.

- Semispinalis thoracis

  □ Origin: Transverse processes of T6 to T10.

  □ Insertion: Spinous processes of C6 to T4.

  □ Innervation: Dorsal primary rami of the thoracic spinal nerves.

  □ Other actions: Contralateral trunk flexion.

- Multifidi

  □ Origin: Articular processes of C4 to C7, transverse processes of T1 to T12, mamillary processes of L1 to L5, sacroiliac ligaments, posterior superior iliac spine, and sacrum.

  □ Insertion: Spinous process of higher vertebrae (2 to 4 and above).

  □ Innervation: Dorsal primary rami of the thoracic and lumbar spinal nerves.

  □ Other actions: Trunk lateral flexion and trunk rotation.

- Rotatores thoracis and lumborum

  - Origin: Transverse processes of the thoracic and lumbar vertebrae.

  - Insertion: Lamina of the next highest vertebrae.

  - Innervation: Dorsal primary rami of the thoracic and lumbar spinal nerves.

  - Other actions: Trunk rotation.

- Interspinalis thoracis and lumborum

  - Origin/Insertion

    - Thoracis: Three pairs between the spinous processes of T1 to T2, T2 to T3, and T11 to T12.

    - Lumbar: Four pairs between the spinous processes of all 5 lumbar vertebrae.

  - Innervation: Dorsal primary rami of the thoracic and lumbar spinal nerves.

  - Other actions: None.

- Intertransversarii thoracis and lumborum

  - Origin/Insertion

    - Thoracis: Eleven pairs between spinous processes of T1 to T12.

    - Lumbar: Four pairs between spinous processes of L1 to L5.

  - Innervation: Dorsal primary rami of the thoracic and lumbar spinal nerves.

  - Other actions: Trunk lateral flexion.

- Quadratus lumborum

  - Origin: Iliolumbar ligaments. Iliac crest and superior borders of the transverse processes of L2 to L5.

  - Insertion: Inferior border of the twelfth rib and transverse processes of L1 to L4.

  - Innervation: Ventral primary rami of L1 to L3.

  - Other actions: Pelvic elevation and trunk lateral flexion.

SECONDARY MOVERS

- Gluteus maximus

ANTI-GRAVITY

- Lumbar

Subject position: Prone with the hands clasped behind the head.

*Alternate position: Prone with pillows under the subject's hips and the hands clasped on the buttocks.

Stabilization: The clinician stabilizes the pelvis and hips.

SUBJECT DIRECTIVE: *"Lift your head and chest up toward the ceiling as high as possible and hold it."* See Figures 2-14 and 2-15.

Figure 2-14. The subject is able to easily reach the endpoint of the movement and hold it against gravity with minimal effort (grade 5/5). For grade 4/5, the subject is able to reach the endpoint of the movement but demonstrates increased effort trying to maintain the position.

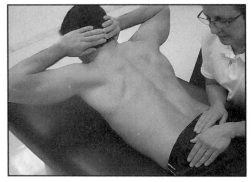

Figure 2-15. The subject is able to complete the maximal range of motion (so that the umbilicus clears the table) with the arms at the subject's sides for a grade of 3/5.

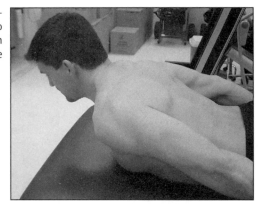

GRAVITY MINIMIZED

- Lumbar

Subject position: Sitting backwards on a chair or on a stool with the hands resting on a tabletop.

Stabilization: Achieved by the weight of the subject on the chair and subject compliance. See Figure 2-16.

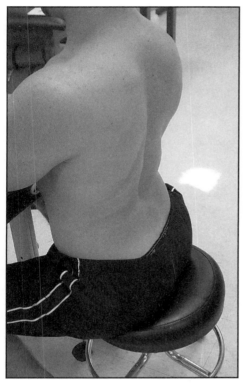

Figure 2-16. The subject extends the lumbar spine, anteriorly tiliting the pelvis, causing increased lumbar lordosis for a grade of 2/5.

- Grades 1/5 to 0/5: See Figure 2-17.

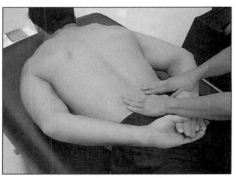

Figure 2-17. The lumbar erector spinae musculature is palpated adjacent to both sides of the spine as the subject attempts to extend.

ANTI-GRAVITY

- Thoracic

Subject position: Prone with the head and upper trunk draped at chest level off the edge of a table with the hands clasped behind the head.

*Alternate position: Prone with pillows under the abdomen and with the hands clasped on the buttocks.

Stabilization: The clinician stabilizes the pelvis and lumbar vertebrae.

SUBJECT DIRECTIVE: *"Lift your head, shoulders, and chest up toward the ceiling as high as possible and hold it."* See Figures 2-18 and 2-19.

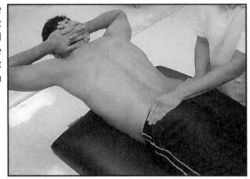

Figure 2-18. The subject is easily able to raise the upper trunk so it is at least horizontal to the tabletop with minimal effort for a grade of 5/5. For grade 4/5, the subject is able to extend the trunk so that it is horizontal to the table level but with some effort.

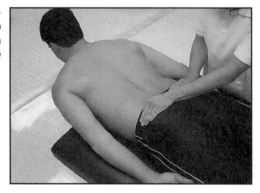

Figure 2-19. The subject is able to complete the maximal range of motion so that the umbilicus clears the table with the arms at the subject's sides for a grade of 3/5.

GRAVITY MINIMIZED

- Thoracic

Subject position: Sitting backwards on a chair with the thoracic spine relaxed and the hands resting on the back of the chair.

Stabilization: Weight of the subject on the chair and subject compliance. See Figure 2-20.

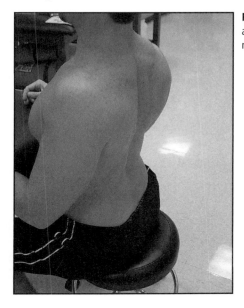

Figure 2-20. The subject extends the thoracic and lumbar spine through the maximal range of motion for a grade of 2/5.

- Grades 1/5 to 0/5: See Figure 2-21.

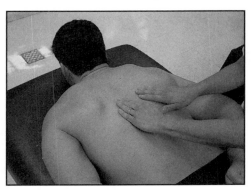

Figure 2-21. The thoracic erector spinae musculature is palpated adjacent to both sides of the spine as the subject attempts to extend.

Substitutions: The subject may use momentum by forcefully pushing the shoulders backwards.

Points of interest: The longissimus is the predominant muscle that is active during all motions of the trunk.

PELVIC ELEVATION

PRIME MOVERS

- Quadratus lumborum

  □ Origin: Superior borders of the transverse processes of L2 to L5.

  □ Insertion: Inferior border of the twelfth rib and transverse processes of L1 to L4.

  □ Innervation: Ventral primary rami of L1 to L3.

  □ Other actions: Lateral trunk flexion to the same side. Stabilizes the twelfth rib during inspiration.

  □ Palpation site: Too deep to be palpated.

SECONDARY MOVERS

- Latissimus dorsi
- Iliocostalis lumborum

ANTI-GRAVITY

Subject position: Standing on a stool or step with the clinician supporting the subject for balance, the test limb hanging free.

Stabilization: The clinician stabilizes the pelvis on the opposite side.

- Grades 5/5 to 4/5: See Figure 2-22.

Figure 2-22. The subject hikes the hip, elevating the pelvis on the side being tested. Resistance is applied in a downward direction on the iliac crest on the tested side, attempting to laterally tilt the pelvis.

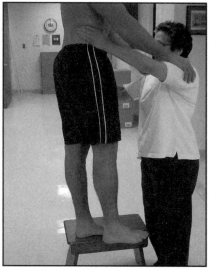

SUBJECT DIRECTIVE: *"Hike your hip up toward your ribs and hold it."*

- Grade 3/5: See Figure 2-23.

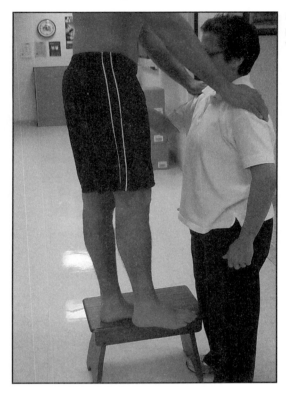

Figure 2-23. The subject hikes the pelvis through the range of motion without resistance.

Substitution: The subject may laterally flex the trunk away from the tested side.

GRAVITY MINIMIZED

Subject position: Supine or prone on a table with the lower extremities in extension.

Stabilization: The subject may hold onto the sides of the table for resistance.

- Grade 2/5: See Figure 2-24.

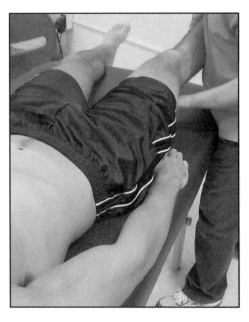

Figure 2-24. The subject hip hikes through the available range of motion.

HIP

FLEXION

ACTIVE RANGE OF MOTION

- 0 to 125 degrees (with the knee flexed)

PRIME MOVERS

- Psoas major

  - Origin: All lumbar vertebral bodies, transverse processes.

  - Insertion: Lesser trochanter of the femur.

  - Innervation: Spinal nerves of L1 to L3.

  - Other actions: Assists with lumbar flexion and lateral flexion of the trunk.

  - Palpation site: Deep into the abdomen inferior to the ribs and superior to the iliac crest, pushing toward the posterior abdominal wall. The subject must be seated and slightly forward flexed to relax the abdominal wall.

- Iliacus

  - Origin: Upper two thirds of the iliac fossa and iliac crest.

  - Insertion: Lesser trochanter of the femur.

  - Innervation: Spinal nerves of L2 to L3.

  - Other actions: None.

  - Palpation site: The iliacus is too deep to palpate accurately.

SECONDARY MOVERS

- Rectus femoris

- Sartorius

- Tensor fasciae latae

- Pectineus

- Adductor brevis

- Adductor magnus (superior fibers)
- Gluteus medius (anterior fibers)

ANTI-GRAVITY

Subject position: Seated on the edge of a table with the arms resting by the sides and the hands on the table for stability.

Stabilization: The clinician stabilizes the opposite side of the pelvis.

- Grades 5/5 to +3/5: See Figure 2-25.

Figure 2-25. Resistance is applied over the distal thigh just proximal to the knee joint in a downward direction.

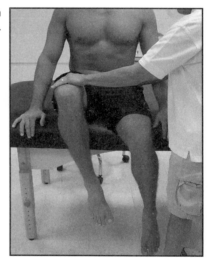

SUBJECT DIRECTIVE: *"Raise your knee up toward the ceiling and hold it. Do not let me push it down."*

- Grades 3/5 to +2/5: See Figure 2-26.

Figure 2-26. The subject is able to flex the hip through the maximal range of motion without resistance.

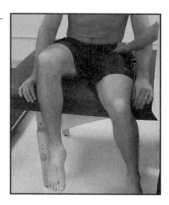

GRAVITY MINIMIZED

Subject position: Sidelying with the tested limb resting on a powder board with the hip in neutral and the knee flexed to 90 degrees or with the clinician supporting the tested limb.

Stabilization: The clinician stabilizes the opposite side of the hip against the table.

- Grades 2/5 to −2/5: See Figure 2-27.

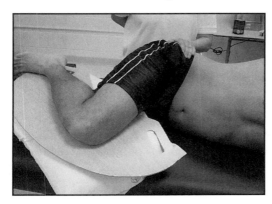

Figure 2-27. The subject is able to flex the hip through the maximal range of motion.

- Grades 1/5 to 0/5: See Figure 2-28.

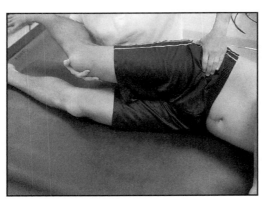

Figure 2-28. The hip flexors are palpated just distal to the inguinal ligament on the medial side of the sartorius as the subject attempts to flex the hip.

Substitutions: The hip may abduct or externally rotate if the sartorius is activated or abduction with internal rotation may occur if the tensor fasciae latae is activated.

Points of interest: Because the psoas major and iliacus share a common insertion and they both flex the hip (and the trunk when the lower extremities are fixed), this muscle group is often referred to as the "iliopsoas." Trauma or retroperitoneal pathology may contribute to weakness of this muscle group.

HIP FLEXION/ABDUCTION/EXTERNAL ROTATION WITH KNEE FLEXION

PRIME MOVERS

- Sartorius

  □ Origin: Anterior superior iliac spine and the upper half of the iliac notch.

  □ Insertion: Proximal aspect of the medial tibia.

  □ Innervation: Femoral nerve (L2 to L3).

  □ Other actions: Assists with flexion of the knee and internal rotation of the tibia when the knee is flexed in non-weight-bearing.

  □ Palpation site: Inferior and slightly medial to the Anterior superior iliac spine.

SECONDARY MOVERS

- All hip and knee flexors
- All hip abductors and external rotators

ANTI-GRAVITY

Subject position: Sitting on the edge of a table with the arms resting by the sides and the hands on the table for stability.

Stabilization: Stabilization is achieved through subject compliance.

- Grades 5/5 to +3/5: See Figure 2-29.

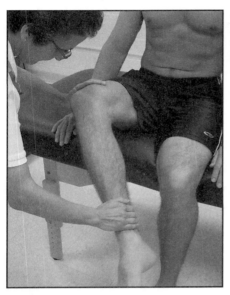

Figure 2-29. Resistance is applied to the medial aspect of the ankle (resisting external rotation of the hip) and to the lateral surface of the thigh proximal to the knee (resisting hip flexion and abduction).

SUBJECT DIRECTIVE: *"Bring the sole of your foot up toward the opposite knee and hold it. Do not let me move your leg."*

- Grades 3/5 to +2/5: See Figure 2-30.

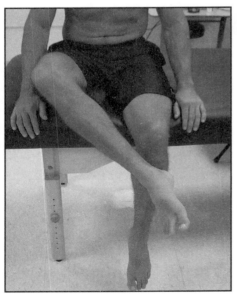

Figure 2-30. The subject is able to move the tested hip through the maximal available range of motion without resistance.

GRAVITY MINIMIZED

Subject position: Supine with the heel of the tested lower leg on the opposite ankle and the nontested lower leg in extension.

Stabilization: Is achieved by the weight of the subject on the table and by subject compliance.

- Grades 2/5 to −2/5: See Figure 2-31.

Figure 2-31. The subject is able to slide the heel of the tested lower leg up toward the opposite knee.

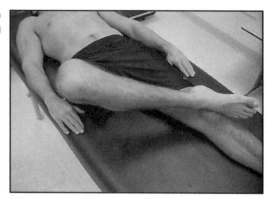

- Grades 1/5 to 0/5: See Figure 2-32.

Figure 2-32. The sartorius may be palpated just inferior to the ASIS at its origin or on the medial side of the thigh as it crosses over the femur.

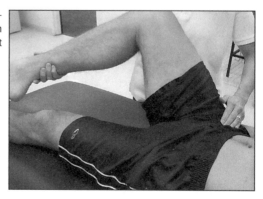

Substitutions: If the hip flexes without abduction or external rotation, the iliopsoas and rectus femoris may be substituting for the sartorius. If the hip flexion and abduction occurs with internal rotation, the tensor fasciae latae is being activated.

Points of interest: The sartorius derives its name from the Latin word *sartor*, which means "tailor" because it helps to initiate the action required to cross the legs when sitting. It is the longest muscle in the body and forms the lateral border of the femoral triangle.

EXTENSION

ACTIVE RANGE OF MOTION

- 0 to 15 degrees (hyperextension)

PRIME MOVERS

- Gluteus maximus

  □ Origin: Posterior gluteal line of the ilium, posterior medial aspect of the iliac crest, dorsal aspect of the sacrum, coccyx, and sacrotubererous ligament.

  □ Insertion: Gluteal tuberosity of the the femur and iliotibial tract.

  □ Innervation: Inferior gluteal nerve (L5 to S2).

  □ Other actions: External rotation of the hip when in extension.

  □ Palpation site: With the hip positioned in external rotation between the sacrum and greater trochanter.

- Semitendinosus

  □ Origin: Upper, inferiomedial impression of the ischial tuberosity (with the tendon of the biceps femoris).

  □ Insertion: Proximal medial shaft of the tibia and pes anserine.

  □ Innervation: Tibial division of the sciatic nerve (L5 to S2).

  □ Other actions: Knee flexion and internal rotation of the tibia when the knee is flexed.

  □ Palpation site: Just proximal to the posterior aspect of the knee joint on the medial side.

- Semimembranosus

  □ Origin: Superolateral aspect of the ischial tuberosity.

  □ Insertion: Posteromedial aspect of the medial tibial condyle.

  □ Innervation: Tibial division of the sciatic nerve (L5 to S2).

- □ Other actions: Knee flexion and internal rotation of the tibia when the knee is flexed.

- □ Palpation site: Just proximal to the posterior aspect of the knee joint on either side of the semitandinosus tendon.

- Biceps femoris

  - □ Origin

    - o Long head: Ischial tuberosity.

    - o Short head: Lateral lip of the linea aspera and the proximal supracondylar line of the femur.

  - □ Insertion

    - o Fibular head: Lateral tibial condyle.

    - o Short head: Peroneal division of the sciatic nerve (L5 to S1).

  - □ Innervation: Long head: Tibial division of the sciatic nerve (L5 to S1).

  - □ Other actions: Knee flexion, external rotation of the tibia when the knee is flexed.

  - □ Palpation site: Along the lateral posterior thigh just proximal to the knee joint.

SECONDARY MOVERS

- Adductor magnus (inferior fibers)

- Gluteus medius (posterior fibers)

ANTI-GRAVITY

Subject position: Prone on a table with the arms by the sides and the lower extremities extended.

*Alternate position: standing with the trunk flexed over a table and with the knee flexed to 90 degrees to isolate the gluteus maximus.

Stabilization: The clinician stabilizes the pelvis against the table.

- Grades 5/5 to +3/5: See Figure 2-33.

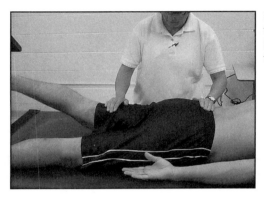

Figure 2-33. Resistance is applied on the posterior thigh just proximal to the knee in a downward direction (toward the floor).

SUBJECT DIRECTIVE: *"Raise your leg as high as you can toward the ceiling and hold it. Do not let me push it down."*

- Grades 3/5 to +2/5: See Figure 2-34.

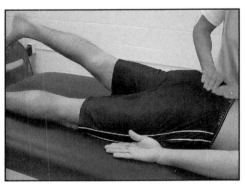

Figure 2-34. The subject is able to raise the limb through the maximal range of motion without resistance.

GRAVITY MINIMIZED

Subject position: Sidelying with the tested limb on top supported on a powder board or by the clinician. The knee is positioned loosely in extension and the bottom hip and knee are flexed for stability.

Stabilization: The clinician stabilizes the pelvis against the table.

- Grades 2/5 to –2/5: See Figure 2-35.

Figure 2-35. The subject extends the hip through the maximal range of motion.

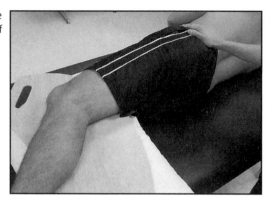

- Grades 1/5 to 0/5: See Figure 2-36.

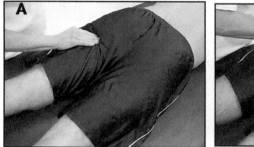 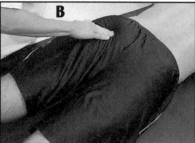

Figure 2-36. (A) The proximal hamstrings are palpated at the ischial tuberosity and (B) the gluteus maximus is palpated deep in the center of the buttock.

Substitutions: The lumbar spine may extend as the subject attempts to extend the hip joint.

Points of interest: The gluteus maximus is the most powerful extensor of the hip. It is primarily active during movements such as stair climbing, rising from a squat to a standing position, and climbing. It is mimimally active during normal gait. If there is weakness of the gluteus maximus, a "gluteus maximus lurch" may result. The hamstrings are significant in maintaining hip extension when in standing.

ABDUCTION

ACTIVE RANGE OF MOTION

- 0 to 45 degrees

PRIME MOVERS

- Gluteus medius

  - Origin: Outer surface of the ilium from the iliac crest and posterior gluteal line above to the anterior gluteal line below.

  - Insertion: Lateral surface of the greater trochanter.

  - Innervation: Superior gluteal nerve (L4 to S1).

  - Other actions: Slight internal rotation of the hip.

  - Palpation site: Just proximal to the greater trochanter and laterally just distal to the iliac crest.

- Gluteus minimus

  - Origin: External surface of the ilium and inferior gluteal line.

  - Insertion: Anterior surface of the greater trochanter.

  - Innervation: Superior gluteal nerve (L4 to S1).

  - Other actions: Slight internal rotation of the hip.

  - Palpation site: The gluteus minimus lies deep to the gluteus maximus and is not palpable.

SECONDARY MOVERS

- Upper fibers of the gluteus maximus
- Tensor fasciae latae
- Obturator internus
- Gemellus superior and inferior
- Sartorius

ANTI-GRAVITY

Subject position: Sidelying with the bottom hip and knee flexed for stability; the tested limb lies on top with the hip and knee extended and in neutral.

Stabilization: The clinician stabilizes the pelvis.

- Grades 5/5 to +3/5: See Figure 2-37.

Figure 2-37. Resistance is applied on the lateral aspect of the thigh just proximal to the knee joint.

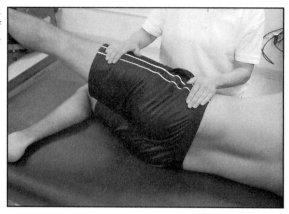

SUBJECT DIRECTIVE: *"Raise your leg up toward the ceiling and hold it. Do not let me push it down."*

- Grades 3/5 to +2/5: See Figure 2-38.

Figure 2-38. The subject abducts the hip through the maximal range of motion without resistance.

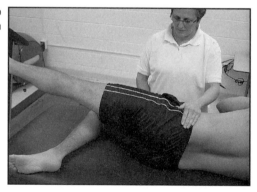

GRAVITY MINIMIZED

Subject position: Supine with the tested limb in extension resting on a smooth surface or supported by the clinician.

Stabilization: The clinician stabilizes the pelvis.

- Grades 2/5 to –2/5: See Figure 2-39.

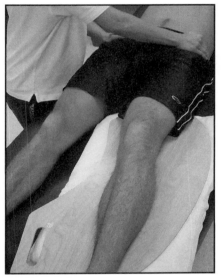

Figure 2-39. The subject abducts the hip through the available range of motion.

- Grades 1/5 to 0/5: See Figure 2-40.

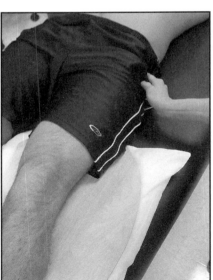

Figure 2-40. The gluteus medius is palpated on the lateral aspect of the hip just superior to the greater trochanter as the subject attempts to abduct the hip.

Substitutions: The subject's pelvis may elevate (hip hike) if the gluteus medius is weak. The tested hip may externally rotate and flex in an attempt to substitute with the hip flexors.

Points of interest: If the gluteus medius and minimus are weak, it will result in a Trendelenburg gait pattern. Only these 2 muscles can stabilize the pelvis during single-limb closed-chain movement.

ABDUCTION FROM A FLEXED HIP

PRIME MOVERS

- Tensor fasciae latae

  □ Origin: Anterior aspect of the outer lip of the iliac crest and the anterior border of the ilium.

  □ Insertion: Lateral aspect of the iliotibial tract, approximately a third of the way down.

  □ Innervation: Superior gluteal nerve (L4 to S1).

  □ Other actions: Assists with internal rotation of the hip, assists with knee extension, and adds stability of the extended knee in standing and during ambulation.

  □ Palpation site: Palpate inferiorly and slightly lateral to the anterior superior iliac spine.

SECONDARY MOVERS

- Gluteus medius

- Gluteus minimus

ANTI-GRAVITY

Subject position: Sidelying with the nontested limb resting in the anatomical position on the table top. The limb to be tested is positioned in approximately 45 degrees of hip flexion with the knee in extension. The foot should be resting on the tabletop.

Stabilization: The clinician stabilizes the pelvis.

- Grades 5/5 to +3/5: See Figure 2-41.

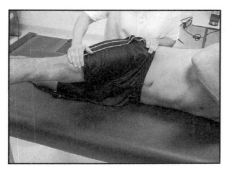

Figure 2-41. Resistance is applied on the lateral aspect of the thigh just proximal to the knee joint while the subject maintains 45 degrees of hip flexion.

SUBJECT DIRECTIVE: *"Raise your leg up toward the ceiling and hold it. Do not let me push it down."*

- Grades 3/5 to +2/5: See Figure 2-42.

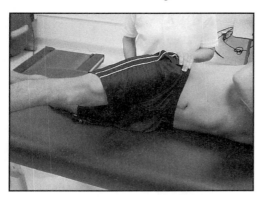

Figure 2-42. The subject abducts the hip through the maximal range of motion, maintaining 45 degrees of hip flexion without resistance.

GRAVITY MINIMIZED

Subject position: Long-sitting on a table with the arms behind the trunk for support, trunk leaning back to put the hips in approximately 45 degrees of flexion. The distal end of the tested limb is supported by the clinician's hand but should not interfere with or assist the movement.

Stabilization: Stabilization is achieved by the weight of the pelvis on the tabletop.

- Grades 2/5: See Figure 2-43.

Figure 2-43. The subject is able to abduct the lower extremity (to 30 degrees) while maintaining 45 degrees of hip flexion.

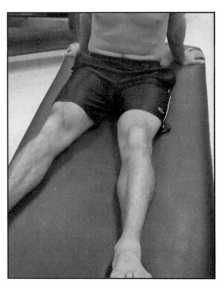

- Grades 1/5 to 0/5: See Figure 2-44.

Figure 2-44. The tensor fascia latae is palpated inferiorly and slightly lateral to the ASIS as the subject attempts to abduct the hip.

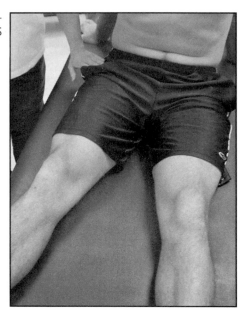

Points of interest: Excessive tightness of the tensor facscia latae bilaterally may result in an anterior pelvis tilt and may contribute to genu valgum. Unilateral tightness of the tensor fascia latae may result in a lateral pelvic tilt.

ADDUCTION

ACTIVE RANGE OF MOTION
- 0 to 30 degrees

PRIME MOVERS
- Adductor magnus

  □ Origin: Inferior ramus of the pubis and ischium and ischial tuberosity.

  □ Insertion: Linea aspera, medial supracondylar line, gluteal tuberosity, and adductor tubercle of the femur.

  □ Innervation: Obturator nerve (L2 to L3) and the tibial division of the sciatic nerve (L2 to L4).

  □ Other actions: Assists with hip flexion/extension and hip internal/external rotation.

  □ Palpation site: Palpate along the middle to lower half of the medial aspect of the thigh.

- Adductor longus

  □ Origin: Anterior surface of the pubis in the angle between the crest and symphysis.

  □ Insertion: Middle third of the linea aspera of the femur.

  □ Innervation: Obturator nerve (L2 to L4).

  □ Other actions: Slight hip flexion.

  □ Palpation site: Palpate just inferior to the pubic arch on the medial aspect of the thigh.

- Adductor brevis

  □ Origin: Inferior aspect of the pubis ramus.

  □ Insertion: Distal pectineal line and proximal portion of the linea aspera of the femur.

  □ Innervation: Obturator nerve (L2 to L4).

- ☐ Other actions: Slight hip flexion.

- ☐ Palpation site: Too deep to palpate.

- Pectineus

  - ☐ Origin: Superior pubic ramus.

  - ☐ Insertion: Line from the lesser trochanter of the femur to the linea aspera.

  - ☐ Innervation: Femoral nerve (L2 to L3) and the obturator nerve (L2 to L3).

  - ☐ Other actions: Hip flexion, slight internal rotation of the hip.

  - ☐ Palpation site: Too deep to palpate.

- Gracilis

  - ☐ Origin: Inferior aspect of the pubic ramus and symphysis.

  - ☐ Insertion: Distal to the medial condyle of the tibia.

  - ☐ Innervation: Obturator nerve (L2 to L3).

  - ☐ Other actions: Assists with knee flexion. Slight internal rotation of the tibia when the knee is in flexion.

  - ☐ Palpation site: Palpate the tendon of the gracilis on the medial aspect of the knee.

SECONDARY MOVERS

- Obturator externus

- Inferior fibers of the gluteus maximus

ANTI-GRAVITY

Subject position: Sidelying with the tested limb resting on the table and the nontested limb supported by the clinician in a position of 25 degrees of abduction.

Stabilization: The pelvis is stabilized by the clinician against the tabletop.

- Grades 5/5 to +3/5: See Figure 2-45.

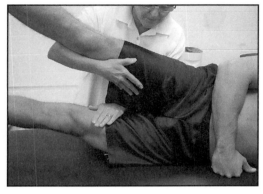

Figure 2-45. Resistance is applied proximal to the knee joint on the medial aspect of the thigh into abduction.

SUBJECT DIRECTIVE: *"Lift your lower leg up so it meets the top leg and hold it. Do not let me push it down."*

- Grades 3/5 to +2/5: See Figure 2-46.

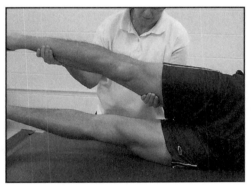

Figure 2-46. The subject adducts the hip through the maximal range of motion without resistance.

GRAVITY MINIMIZED

Subject position: Supine with the tested limb supported by the clinician in a slight amount of abduction and the nontested limb resting in 25 degrees of abduction.

Stabilization: Stabilization is achieved through the weight of the pelvis/ trunk on the tabletop.

■ Grades 2/5 to –2/5: See Figure 2-47.

Figure 2-47. The subject adducts the hip through the maximal range of motion.

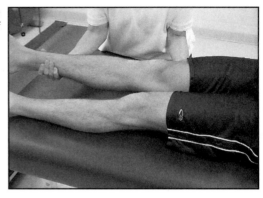

■ Grades 1/5 to 0/5: See Figure 2-48.

Figure 2-48. The adductor longus is palpated on the medial aspect of the thigh just inferior to the pubic arch, the adductor magnus is palpable along the medial aspect of the thigh (middle to lower portion), and the gracilis can be palpated along the medial aspect of the knee as the subject attempts to adduct the limb.
(Shown: Palpating the adductor magnus.)

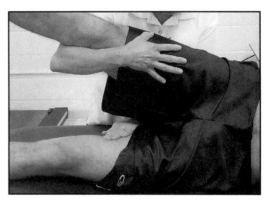

Substitutions: The subject may internally rotate the hip in an attempt to use the hip flexors to substitute for the hip adductors. The subject may externally rotate the hip in an attempt to substitute the hamstrings for the hip adductors during the movement.

Points of interest: It is not possible to isolate individual muscles during testing, so the adductors must be tested as a group. Depending on whether or not the femur is in flexion or extension, the adductors may assist during internal or external rotary movements of the hip.

INTERNAL (MEDIAL) ROTATION

ACTIVE RANGE OF MOTION

- 0 to 45 degrees (with the hip flexed)

- 0 to 30 degrees (with the hip extended)

PRIME MOVERS

- Gluteus medius (anterior fibers)

  - Origin: Outer surface of the ilium from the iliac crest and posterior gluteal line above to the anterior gluteal line below.

  - Insertion: Lateral surface of the greater trochanter.

  - Innervation: Superior gluteal nerve (L4 to S1).

  - Other actions: Hip abduction.

  - Palpation site: Just proximal to the greater trochanter and laterally just distal to the iliac crest.

- Gluteus minimus (anterior fibers)

  - Origin: External surface of the ilium and inferior gluteal line.

  - Insertion: Anterior surface of the greater trochanter.

  - Innervation: Superior gluteal nerve (L4 to S1).

  - Other actions: Hip abduction.

  - Palpation site: The gluteus minimus lies deep to the gluteus maximus and is not palpable.

- Tensor fasciae latae

  - Origin: Anterior aspect of the outer lip of the iliac crest and the anterior border of the ilium.

  - Insertion: Lateral aspect of the iliotibial tract, approximately two thirds of the way down.

  - Innervation: Superior gluteal nerve (L4 to S1).

  - Other actions: Hip flexion, abduction, and knee extension. It also adds stability to the extended knee when standing and during ambulation.

  - Palpation site: Palpate inferiorly and slightly lateral to the anterior superior iliac spine.

SECONDARY MOVERS

- Semitendinosus

- Semimembranosus

- Adductor magnus

- Adductor longus

ANTI-GRAVITY

Subject position: Sitting, with the knees flexed over the edge of a table.

Stabilization: The clinician stabilizes the distal thigh and the medial side of the knee joint.

- Grades 5/5 to +3/5: See Figure 2-49.

Figure 2-49. Resistance is applied to the lower leg just proximal to the lateral malleolus into external rotation.

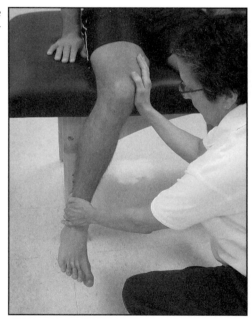

SUBJECT DIRECTIVE: *"Rotate your lower leg away from your other leg and hold it. Do not let me push it in."*

- Grades 3/5 to +2/5: See Figure 2-50.

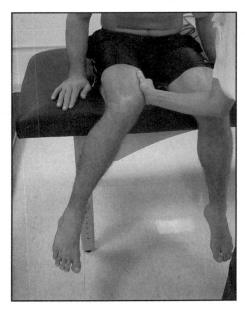

Figure 2-50. The subject internally rotates the tested leg through the maximal range of motion without resistance.

GRAVITY MINIMIZED

Subject position: Supine with the knees extended and the tested hip in slight external rotation.

Stabilization: The clinician stabilizes the pelvis against the tabletop.

- Grades 2/5 to −2/5: See Figure 2-51.

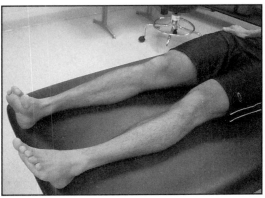

Figure 2-51. The subject internally rotates the hip through the available range of motion.

- Grades 1/5 to 0/5: See Figure 2-52.

Figure 2-52. Only the anterior and middle fibers of the gluteus medius are palpable laterally below the crest of the ilium.

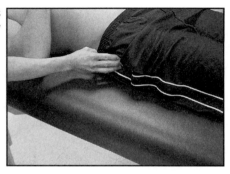

Substitutions: The subject may lift the pelvis off the table on the tested side, extend the knee/hip, or adduct the hip during testing.

EXTERNAL (LATERAL) ROTATION

ACTIVE RANGE OF MOTION

- 0 to 45 degrees (with the hip flexed)

- 0 to 30 degrees (with the hip extended)

PRIME MOVERS

- Obturator externus

  □ Origin: External surface of the obturator membrane, inferior ramus of the pubis and ischium.

  □ Insertion: Trochanteric fossa of the femur.

  □ Innervation: Obturator nerve (L3 to L4).

  □ Other actions: None.

  □ Palpation site: Too deep to palpate.

- Obturator internus

  □ Origin: Internal margin of the obturator foramen, ischial ramus, and obturator membrane.

  □ Insertion: Medial aspect of the greater trochanter of the femur.

- Innervation: Obturator nerve (L3 to L4).

- Other actions: None.

- Palpation site: Too deep to palpate.

- **Piriformis**

  - Origin: Anterior surface of the sacrum, gluteal surface of the ilium near the posterior inferior iliac spine, sacrotuberous ligament, capsule of the sacroiliac joint/border of the greater sciatic foramen.

  - Insertion: Superior surface of the greater trochanter of the femur.

  - Innervation: Sacral nerve (S1 to S2).

  - Other actions: None.

  - Palpation site: Too deep to accurately palpate.

- **Superior gemellus**

  - Origin: Dorsal surface of the ischial spine.

  - Insertion: Medial surface of the greater trochanter.

  - Innervation: Obturator nerve/sacral plexus (L5 to S1).

  - Other actions: None.

  - Palpation site: Too deep to palpate.

- **Inferior gemellus**

  - Origin: Ischial tuberosity.

  - Insertion: Medial surface of the greater trochanter of the femur, blending with the tendon of the obturator internus.

  - Innervation: Obturator nerve/sacral plexus (L5 to S1).

  - Other actions: None.

  - Palpation site: Too deep to palpate.

- **Quadratus femoris**

  - Origin: Lateral aspect of the ischial tuberosity.

  - Insertion: Intertrochanteric crest.

  - Innervation: Sacral plexus (L5 to S1).

□ Other actions: None.

□ Palpation site: Too deep to palpate.

SECONDARY MOVERS

- Sartorius

- Long head of the biceps femoris

- Posterior aspect of the gluteus medius

- Psoas major

- Adductor magnus

- Adductor longus

- Popliteus (with a fixed tibia)

ANTI-GRAVITY

Subject position: Sitting, with the knees flexed over the edge of a table.

Stabilization: The clinician stabilizes the distal thigh/knee joint on the lateral side.

- Grades 5/5 to +3/5: See Figure 2-53.

Figure 2-53. Resistance is applied to the lower leg just proximal to the medial malleolus into internal rotation.

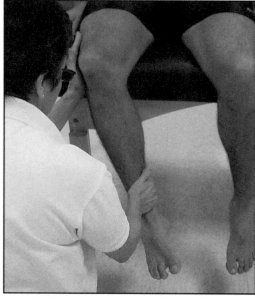

SUBJECT DIRECTIVE: *"Rotate your lower leg toward your other leg and hold it. Do not let me push it out."*

- Grades 3/5 to +2/5: See Figure 2-54.

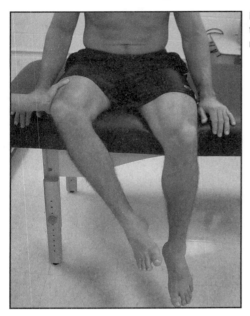

Figure 2-54. The subject externally rotates the tested hip through the maximal range of motion without resistance.

GRAVITY MINIMIZED

Subject position: Supine with the knees extended and the tested hip in slight internal rotation.

Stabilization: The clinician stabilizes the pelvis against the tabletop.

- Grades 2/5 to –2/5: See Figure 2-55.

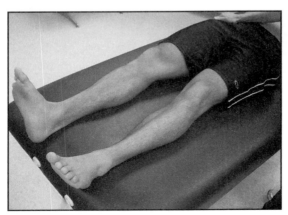

Figure 2-55. The subject externally rotates the hip through the maximal range of motion.

Because the external rotators are too deep to palpate (except for the gluteus maximus), a grade of 1/5 should be assigned if any contractile activity is observed. If the clinician is in doubt that the movement seen is a result of the lateral rotators contracting, a grade of 0/5 is appropriate.

Substitutions: In the anti-gravity position, the subject may lift the contracting buttock off the table, flex the knee, and abduct/adduct the hip during testing to substitute for hip external rotation.

Points of interest: The sciatic nerve runs between the lateral rotators of the femur and piriformis and may become entrapped or compressed by the piriformis, causing buttock and/or posterior thigh pain. These small muscles may be remembered in anatomical order from superior to inferior by the acronym "Piece Goods Often Go On Quilts" (Piriformis, Gemellus superior, Obturator internus, Gemellus inferior, Obturator externus, and Quadratus femoris).

KNEE

FLEXION

ACTIVE RANGE OF MOTION

- 0 to 120 degrees (with the hip in extension)

- 0 to 135 degrees (with the hip in flexion)

PRIME MOVERS

- Biceps femoris

  □ Origin

    o Long head: Ischial tuberosity and sacrotuberous ligament.

    o Short head: Linea aspera of the femur, lateral/proximal supra-condylar line of the femur.

  □ Insertion

    o Long and short heads: Head of the fibula and lateral tibial condyle.

  □ Innervation

    o Long head: Tibial division of the sciatic nerve (L5 to S2).

    o Short head: Peroneal division of the sciatic nerve (L5 to S2).

  □ Other actions: Hip extension and external rotation of the tibia when the knee is flexed.

  □ Palpation site: Along the lateral/posterior thigh, immediately proximal to the knee joint.

- Semitendinosus

  □ Origin: Ischial tuberosity.

  □ Insertion: Proximal/medial shaft of the tibia; pes anserine.

  □ Innervation: Tibial division of the sciatic nerve (L5 to S2).

  □ Other actions: Hip extension and internal rotation of the tibia when the knee is flexed.

  □ Palpation site: Just proximal to the posterior knee joint line on the medial side.

- Semimembranosus

  □ Origin: Ischial tuberosity.

  □ Insertion: Posteromedial aspect of the medial tibial condyle.

  □ Innervation: Tibial division of the sciatic nerve (L5 to S2).

  □ Other actions: Hip extension and internal rotation of the tibia when the knee is flexed.

  □ Palpation site: Just proximal to the posterior knee joint line on both sides of the semitendinosus tendon with the knee in slight flexion (between 0 and 45 degrees).

SECONDARY MOVERS

- Gracilis
- Tensor fasciae latae
- Sartorius
- Popliteus
- Gastrocnemius
- Plantaris

ANTI-GRAVITY

Subject position: Prone with the tested hip in neutral rotation and the knee flexed to approximately 45 degrees.

Stabilization: The clinician stabilizes the thigh against the table.

- Grades 5/5 to +3/5: See Figure 2-56.

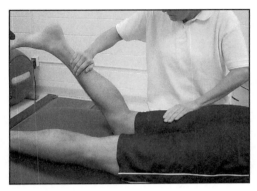

Figure 2-56. Resistance is applied just proximal to the posterior aspect of the ankle joint into knee extension.

SUBJECT DIRECTIVE: *"Bend your knee and hold it. Do not let me push it down."*

To test the medial hamstrings (semitendinosus/semimembranosus), the tibia should be maintained in internal rotation. To test the lateral hamstring (biceps femoris), the tibia should be maintained in external rotation.

- Grades 3/5 to +2/5: See Figure 2-57.

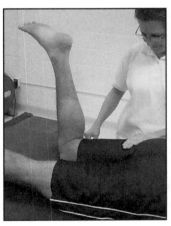

Figure 2-57. The subject flexes the knee through the range of motion and is able to hold the end range position against gravity.

GRAVITY MINIMIZED

Subject position: Sidelying with the tested limb on top and either supported by the clinician or resting on a powder board. The lower limb is slightly flexed for stability.

Stabilization: The clinician stabilizes the thigh to prevent the hip from flexing during testing.

- Grades 2/5 to –2/5: See Figure 2-58.

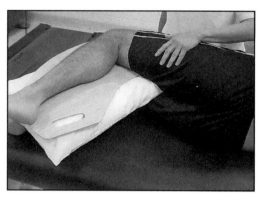

Figure 2-58. The subject flexes the knee through the maximal range of motion.

- Grades 1/5 to 0/5: See Figure 2-59.

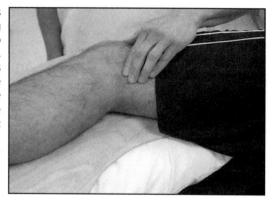

Figure 2-59. The tendon of the biceps femoris is visible and palpated along the posterior thigh just proximal to the posteriolateral aspect of the knee. The tendons of the semitendinosus and semimembranosus are visible and palpated just proximal to the posteromedial aspect of the knee joint as the subject attempts to flex the knee.
(Shown: Palpating the biceps femoris.)

Substitutions: The hip may abduct/adduct or flex as the subject attempts to flex the knee because of the actions of the gracilis and sartorius. In addition, the gastrocnemius may cause plantar flexion of the ankle during testing.

*If the lateral hamstring is stronger than the medial hamstrings, the tibia will externally rotate during testing. If the medial hamstrings are stronger than the lateral hamstring, the tibia will internally rotate during testing.

EXTENSION

ACTIVE RANGE OF MOTION

- 120 to 0 degrees (from knee flexion with the hip extended)
- 135 to 0 degrees (from knee flexion with the hip flexed)

PRIME MOVERS

- Rectus femoris

  - □ Origin: Anterior inferior iliac spine and the superior rim of the acetabulum.

  - □ Insertion: Tibial tuberosity via the patellar ligament.

  - □ Innervation: Femoral nerve (L2 to L4).

  - □ Other actions: Hip flexion.

  - □ Palpation site: Between the sartorius and tensor fascia latae of the proximal thigh.

- Vastus intermedius

  - □ Origin: Upper two thirds of the anterior and lateral shaft of the femur and the distal half of the linea aspera.

  - □ Insertion: Tibial tuberosity via the patellar ligment.

  - □ Innervation: Femoral nerve (L2 to L4).

  - □ Other actions: None.

  - □ Palpation site: Too deep to palpate.

- Vastus medialis

  - □ Origin: Medial lip of the linea aspera of the femur, distal inter-trochanteric line, origin of the vastus medialis oblique, proximal supracondylar line, and tendon of the adductor magnus.

  - □ Insertion: Tibial tuberosity via the patellar ligament.

  - □ Innervation: Femoral nerve (L2 to L4).

  - □ Other actions: None.

  - □ Palpation site: Medial aspect to the thigh, just proximal to the patella.

- Vastus lateralis

  - □ Origin: Lateral lip of the linea aspera of the femur, proximal aspect of the intertrochanteric line, inferior greater trochanter, lateral lip of the gluteal tuberosity.

  - □ Insertion: Tibial tuberosity via the patellar ligament.

  - □ Innervation: Femoral nerve (L2 to L4).

  - □ Other actions: None.

  - □ Palpation site: Lateral aspect of the thigh.

SECONDARY MOVERS

- Tensor fascia latae

ANTI-GRAVITY

Subject position: Sitting with both knees flexed to 90 degrees and hanging freely over the edge of a table.

Stabilization: The weight of the trunk and thigh provide stabilization for the lower leg.

- Grades 5/5 to +3/5: See Figure 2-60.

Figure 2-60. Resistance is applied just proximal to the ankle joint on the anterior aspect of the lower leg.

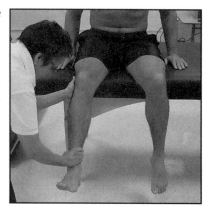

SUBJECT DIRECTIVE: *"Straighten out your knee and hold it up. Do not let me push it down."*

- Grades 3/5 to +2/5: See Figure 2-61.

Figure 2-61. The subject is able to extend the knee through the maximal range of motion and is able to hold the end range position without resistance.

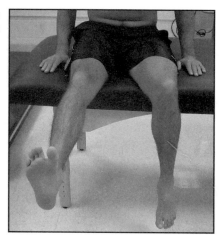

GRAVITY MINIMIZED

Subject postion: Sidelying with the tested limb on top resting on a powder board with the knee flexed to 90 degrees. The bottom knee should be slightly flexed for improved stability.

Stabilization: Stabilization is achieved through the weight of the lower limb, pelvis, and trunk lying against the table.

■ Grades 2/5 to –2/5: See Figure 2-62.

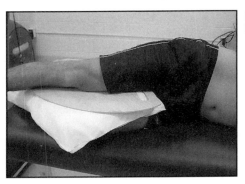

Figure 2-62. The subject extends the tested knee through the maximal range of motion.

■ Grades 1/5 to 0/5: See Figure 2-63.

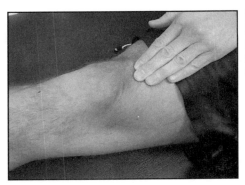

Figure 2-63. With the subject lying supine, the distal aspect of the quadriceps muscle group is palpated just proximal to the patella as the subject attempts to contract the anterior thigh.

Substitutions: The subject may attempt to internally rotate or extend the hip, allowing the knee to passively move into extension.

Points of interest: The rectus femoris is the only muscle in the quadriceps femoris group that crosses both the hip and knee joints. Its actions move the lower extremity forward while ambulating and extend the knee when performing a closed chain activity such as jumping. Weakness of the quadriceps group impairs the ability to move sit to stand, ambulate uphill, or stair climb.

ANKLE

DORSIFLEXION/INVERSION

PRIME MOVERS

- Tibialis anterior

  □ Origin: Distal to the lateral tibial condyle, proximal/lateral half of the surface of the tibial shaft, and medial aspect of the fibula and the anterior interosseus membrane.

  □ Insertion: Medial and plantar surface of the medial cuneiform bone and base of the first metatarsal.

  □ Innervation: Deep peroneal nerve (L4 to S1).

  □ Other actions: None.

  □ Palpation site: Along the lateral side of the tibia and as the tendon crosses the dorsum of the foot from the medial to lateral side.

SECONDARY MOVERS

- Peroneus tertius

- Extensor digitorum longus

- Extensor hallucis longus

ANTI-GRAVITY

Subject position: Sitting with the knee flexed over the edge of a table with the ankle/foot in a relaxed position.

*Alternate position: The subject may lie in supine with the ankle/foot hanging freely over the edge of a table.

Stabilization: The thigh is stabilized against the tabletop while the clinician stabilizes the lower leg.

- Grades 5/5 to +3/5: See Figure 2-64.

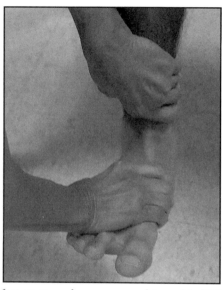

Figure 2-64. Resistance is applied to the medial/dorsal surface of the forefoot into plantar flexion and eversion.

SUBJECT DIRECTIVE: *"Move your foot up toward your nose and in and hold it there. Do not let me push it down."*

- Grades 3/5 to +2/5: See Figure 2-65.

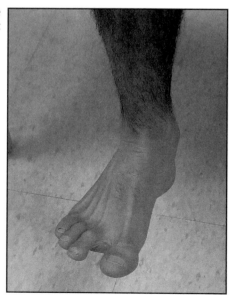

Figure 2-65. The subject dorsiflexes the ankle through the maximal range of motion without resistance.

GRAVITY MINIMIZED

Subject position: Sidelying with the tested limb/ankle on top resting on a powder board or smooth surface.

- Grades 2/5 to –2/5: See Figure 2-66.

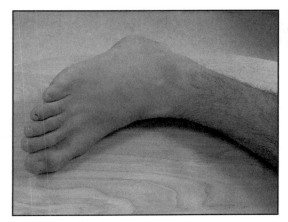

Figure 2-66. The subject dorsiflexes the ankle through the maximal range of motion.

- Grades 1/5 to 0/5: See Figure 2-67.

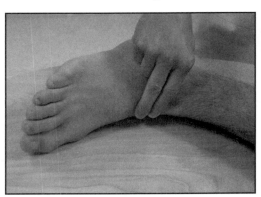

Figure 2-67. The tendon of the tibialis anterior is palpated as it crosses the dorsum of the foot as the subject attempts to dorsiflex the ankle.

Substitutions: The extensor digitorum longus and extensor hallucis longus may contract, causing toe extension. The tibialis posterior will cause inversion without dorsiflexion and the extensor digitorum longus will cause dorsiflexion with eversion.

PLANTAR FLEXION

ACTIVE RANGE OF MOTION

- 0 to 45 degrees

PRIME MOVERS

- Gastrocnemius

  □ Origin

    o Medial head: Popliteal surface of the medial femoral condyle and capsule of the knee joint.

    o Lateral head: Lateral surface of the lateral femoral condyle and capsule of the knee joint.

  □ Insertion: Posterior surface of the calcaneus via the Achilles' tendon.

  □ Innervation: Tibial nerve (S1 to S2).

  □ Other actions: Flexion of the knee.

  □ Palpation site: Immediately distal to the posterior knee joint line.

- Plantaris

  □ Origin: Lateral supracondylar line of the femur.

  □ Insertion: Medial aspect of the posterior part of the calcaneus via the Achilles' tendon.

  □ Innervation: Tibial nerve (S1 to S2).

  □ Other actions: Slight knee flexion.

  □ Palpation site: Too deep to palpate.

- Soleus

  □ Origin: Head of the fibula, proximal third of the fibular shaft, soleal line, and mid-shaft of the posterior/medial border of the tibia.

  □ Insertion: Medial side of the posterior surface of the calcaneus via the Achilles' tendon.

  □ Innervation: Tibial nerve (S1 to S2).

  □ Other actions: None.

  □ Palpation site: Bilaterally distal to the belly of the gastrocnemius.

SECONDARY MOVERS

- Tibialis posterior

- Peroneus longus

- Peroneus brevis

- Flexor digitorum longus

- Flexor hallucis longus

ANTI-GRAVITY

Subject position: Single-leg standing on the tested limb with the knee in maximal extension. The opposite foot should be off the floor and the subject should balance him- or herself with 1 to 2 fingers on a tabletop or countertop.

Stabilization: Provided with 1 to 2 fingers on a tabletop or countertop.

- Grades 5/5 to 3/5: See Figures 2-68 and 2-69.

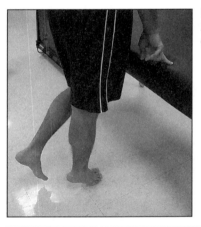

Figure 2-68. The subject easily completes at least 25 heel raises through the maximal range of motion with good form.

*Grade 4/5 is assigned if the subject is able to perform 10 to 24 heel raises through the maximal range of motion with good form and with no effort. Grade 3/5 is assigned if the subject is able to perform 1 to 9 heel raises through the maximal range of motion with good form and with no effort. The grade is dropped to the next lower level if subject is unable to complete the maximal range of motion on any given repetition.

SUBJECT DIRECTIVE: *"Stand on your right leg and push up onto your toes. Please repeat this as many times as you can until I tell you to stop."*

Figure 2-69. To test the soleus individually, the subject should stand on the tested limb with the knee in slight flexion.

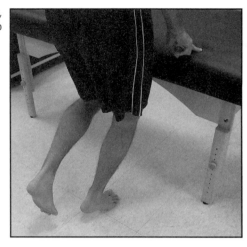

GRAVITY MINIMIZED

Subject position: Prone with the tested foot/ankle off the edge of a table.

Stabilization: Provided by the weight of the thigh/pelvis on the tabletop.

- Grade 2/5: See Figure 2-70A.

- Grade +2/5: See Figure 2-70B.

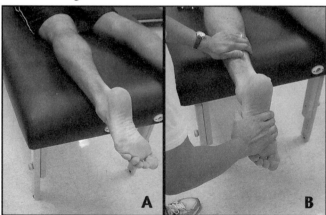

Figures 2-70A and B. The subject is able to plantarflex the ankle through the maximal range of motion.

A grade of +2/5 is assigned if the subject can plantarflex through the maximal range of motion and hold it against maximal resistance. A grade of −2/5 is assigned if the subject completes partial range of motion without resistance.

■ Grades 1/5 to 0/5: See Figure 2-71.

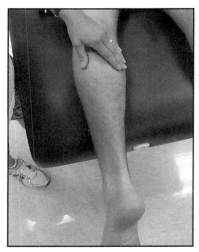

Figure 2-71. The gastrocnemius muscle is palpated at mid-calf with the thumb and fingers on either side of the muscle belly (above the soleus) and the soleus is palpated on the posterolateral surface of the distal calf as the subject attempts to plantarflex the ankle. (Shown: Palpating the gastrocnemius.)

Substitutions: When standing, the subject may lean forward during testing, allowing the heel to passively raise off the floor. When lying in prone, substitution by the peroneus longus and brevis will cause the foot to move into eversion, and substitution by the tibialis posterior will cause the foot to invert. Substitution by the flexor hallucis longus and flexor digitorum longus will result in flexion of the toes and plantar flexion of the foot.

Points of interest: Although the gastrocnemius crosses both the knee and ankle joint, it can only act on the knee and ankle separately, not simultaneously. The word *soleus* is Latin for sole, which is a flat fish. This muscle lies deep to the gastrocnemius and is the stronger plantar flexor of the two. They are responsible for raising the heel during jumping or running.

INVERSION

ACTIVE RANGE OF MOTION
■ 0 to 30 degrees

PRIME MOVERS
■ Tibialis posterior

  □ Origin: Posterior surface of the shaft of the tibia, proximal two thirds of the posterior aspect of the fibula, and the posterior interosseous membrane.

  □ Insertion: Tuberosity of the navicular; plantar surface of the cuneiform bones; plantar surface of the basse of the second, third, and fourth metatarsals; the cuboid and sustentaculum tali.

□ Innervation: Tibial nerve (L4 to L5).

□ Other actions: Plantar flexion of the ankle.

□ Palpation site: Between the medial malleolus and navicular.

SECONDARY MOVERS

- Tibialis anterior

- Flexor digitorum longus

- Flexor hallucis longus

- Soleus

- Extensor hallucis longus

ANTI-GRAVITY

Subject position: Sidelying with the tested foot and ankle over the edge of a table.

Stabilization: The lower limb is stabilized by the clinician against the tabletop.

- Grades 5/5 to +3/5: See Figure 2-72.

Figure 2-72. Resistance is applied to the medial border of the forefoot into eversion and dorsiflexion.

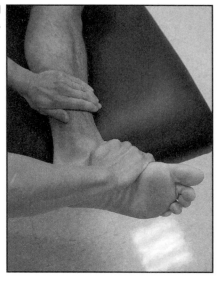

SUBJECT DIRECTIVE: *"Move your foot down and in and hold it. Do not let me push it out."*

- Grades 3/5 to +2/5: See Figure 2-73.

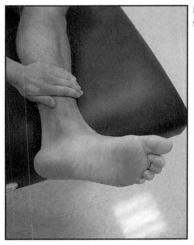

Figure 2-73. The subject is able to invert the foot through the maximal range of motion without resistance.

GRAVITY MINIMIZED

Subject position: Supine with the tested foot/ankle over the edge of a table.

Stabilization: The lower limb is stabilized by the clinician against the table-top.

- Grades 2/5 to −2/5: See Figure 2-74.

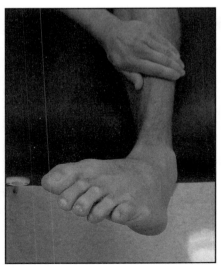

Figure 2-74. The subject is able to invert the foot through the maximal range of motion.

■ Grades 1/5 to 0/5: See Figure 2-75.

Figure 2-75. The posterior tibialis tendon is palpated as it crosses between the medial malleolus and navicular as the subject attempts to invert the ankle.

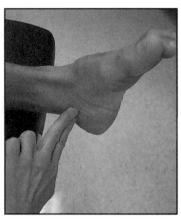

Substitutions: The tibialis anterior may cause dorsiflexion as the ankle inverts and the toe flexors may contribute to inversion and plantar flexion of the foot.

Points of interest: The tibialis posterior is the deepest of the posterior calf muscles whose tendons course around the medial malleolus (the others being the flexor digitorum longus and flexor hallucis longus), otherwise known as "Tom, Dick, and Harry." In addition to its primary actions, it is a major component of the longitudinal arch of the foot.

EVERSION

ACTIVE RANGE OF MOTION
■ 0 to 25 degrees

PRIME MOVERS
■ Peroneus longus

  □ Origin: Lateral condyle of the tibia, head, and proximal two thirds of the lateral surface of the fibula.

  □ Insertion: Lateral aspect of the first cuneiform bone and the base of the first metatarsal.

  □ Innervation: Superficial peroneal nerve (L5 to S1).

  □ Other actions: Slight plantar flexion of the ankle.

  □ Palpation site: Just distal to the lateral malleolus as it runs to the plantar surface of the foot.

- Peroneus brevis

  □ Origin: Distal two thirds of the lateral fibular shaft.

  □ Insertion: Tuberosity of the fifth metatarsal.

  □ Innervation: Superficial peroneal nerve (L5 to S1).

  □ Other actions: Slight plantar flexion of the anke.

  □ Palpation site: Just distal to the lateral malleolus as it runs anteriorly toward the fifth metatarsal.

- Peroneus tertius

  □ Origin: Lateral slip from the extensor digitorum longus.

  □ Insertion: Tuberosity of the fifth metatarsal.

  □ Innervation: Deep peroneal nerve (L5 to S1).

  □ Other actions: Slight dorsiflexion of the ankle.

  □ Palpation site (if present): Laterally on the forefoot toward the fifth metatarsal.

SECONDARY MOVERS

- Extensor digitorum longus

ANTI-GRAVITY

Subject position: Sidelying with the tested foot and ankle over the edge of a table.

Stabilization: The lower limb is stabilized by the clinician against the tabletop.

- Grades 5/5 to +3/5: See Figure 2-76.

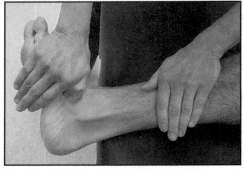

Figure 2-76. Resistance is applied to the lateral border of the forefoot into inversion and plantar flexion.

SUBJECT DIRECTIVE: *"Move your foot up and out and hold it. Do not let me push it down."*

- Grades 3/5 to +2/5: See Figure 2-77.

Figure 2-77. The subject is able to evert the foot through the maximal range of motion without resistance.

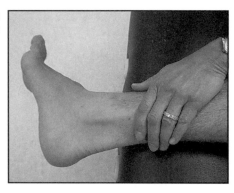

GRAVITY MINIMIZED

Subject position: Supine with the tested foot/ankle over the edge of a table.

Stabilization: The lower limb is stabilized by the clinician against the table-top.

- Grades 2/5 to –2/5: See Figure 2-78.

Figure 2-78. The subject is able to evert the foot through the maximal range of motion.

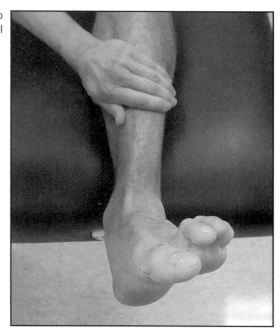

- Grades 1/5 to 0/5: See Figure 2-79.

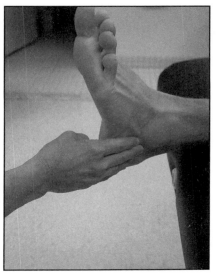

Figure 2-79. The tendons of the peroneus longus and brevis are palpated just distal to the lateral malleolus as the subject attempts to evert the ankle/foot.

Substitutions: Substitution by the extensor digitorum may cause the ankle to dorsiflex. The flexor digitorum may contract to cause eversion with some plantar flexion of the foot.

Points of interest: The actions of the ankle evertors are critical in keeping the ankle stable during activities taking place on uneven surfaces. The peroneus tertius acts to place the foot flat on the ground by raising the lateral border of the foot. This group may also be known as the "fibularis" longus, brevis, and tertius.

GREAT TOE

Note: Because gravity is not a significant factor during testing of the toes, the format used for grading muscle strength deviates from the standard grading system applied to other muscle groups; half grades are not assigned.

FLEXION

ACTIVE RANGE OF MOTION

- 0 to 45 degrees (metatarsophalangeal [MTP] flexion)

- 0 to 90 degrees (interphalangeal [IP] flexion)

PRIME MOVERS

- Flexor hallucis brevis

  □ Origin

    o Lateral head: Plantar surface of the cuboid and lateral cuneiform bone.

    o Medial head: Medial intermuscular septum and the tibialis posterior tendon.

  □ Insertion

    o Lateral head: Proximal phalanx of the hallux (on both sides of the base) joining with the adductor hallucis.

    o Medial head: Proximal phalanx of the hallux (on both sides of the base) joining with the abductor hallucis.

  □ Innervation: Medial plantar nerve (S2).

  □ Other actions: None.

  □ Palpation site: Along the medial arch of the foot, adjacent to the first metatarsal head.

- Flexor hallucis longus

  □ Origin: Distal two thirds of the posterior aspect of the fibular shaft.

  □ Insertion: Base of the distal phalanx of the great toe.

  □ Innervation: Tibial nerve (L5 to S2).

  □ Other actions: Slight plantar flexion of the ankle.

  □ Palpation site: Palpate the tendon as it crosses the plantar surface of the proximal phalanx of the great toe.

SECONDARY MOVERS

- Adductor hallucis

- Abductor hallucis

Grades 5/5 (normal), 4/5 (good), 3/5 (fair), and 2/5 (poor)

Subject position: Sitting or supine with the tested knee in extension and the ankle and foot in neutral and resting on a table.

Stabilization: The foot is stabilized by the clinician.

- Grades 5/5 to 4/5: See Figure 2-80.

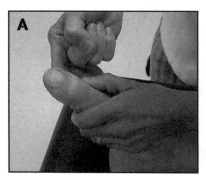
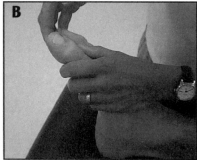

Figure 2-80. Resistance is applied on the plantar surfaces of the (A) proximal and (B) distal phalanx of the great toe to test the MTP and IP joints, respectively.

SUBJECT DIRECTIVE: *"Curl your big toe over my finger and hold it. Do not let me straighten it out."*

- Grade 3/5: See Figure 2-81.

Figure 2-81. The subject is able to flex the great toe through the maximal range of motion but is unable to maintain the position against resistance.

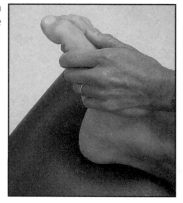

Grade 2/5 is assigned for partial range of motion.

GRADES 1/5 (TRACE) AND 0/5 (ZERO)

- Grades 1/5 to 0/5: See Figure 2-82.

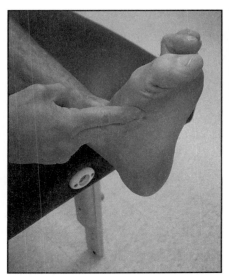

Figure 2-82. The flexor hallucis brevis is palpated along the medial arch of the foot, adjacent to the first metatarsal head and the flexor hallucis longus tendon is palpated as it crosses the plantar aspect of the proximal phalanx as the subject attempts to flex the great toe. (Shown: Palpating the flexor hallucis brevis.)

Points of interest: The flexor hallucis is active during walking and running by flexing the great toe to push off the ground.

EXTENSION

ACTIVE RANGE OF MOTION

- 45 to 0 degrees (MTP extension)
- 0 to 90 degrees (MTP hyperextension)
- 90 to 0 degrees (IP extension)

PRIME MOVERS

- Extensor hallucis brevis
  - □ Origin: Distal superolateral surface of the calcaneus.
  - □ Insertion: Dorsal surface of the proximal phalanx.
  - □ Innervation: Deep peroneal nerve (S1 to S2).

- ☐ Other actions: None.

- ☐ Palpation site: Dorsolateral surface of the foot.

- Extensor hallucis longus

  - ☐ Origin: Middle half of the medial aspect of the fibular shaft.

  - ☐ Insertion: Base of the distal phalanx of the great toe.

  - ☐ Innervation: Deep peroneal nerve (L5 to S1).

  - ☐ Other actions: Slight dorsiflexion of the ankle.

  - ☐ Palpation site: Dorsum of the foot, lateral to the tibialis anterior tendon as it crosses the dorsal aspect of the first metatarsal.

SECONDARY MOVERS

- None

Grades 5/5 (normal), 4/5 (good), 3/5 (fair), and 2/5 (poor)

Subject position: Sitting or supine with both lower limbs extended and with the ankle and foot in neutral resting on a table.

Stabilization: The clinician stabilizes the foot and first metatarsal bone.

- Grades 5/5 to 4/5: See Figure 2-83.

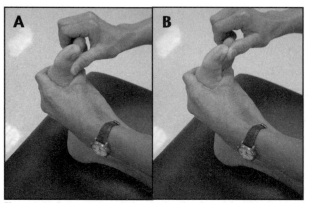

Figure 2-83. Resistance is applied to the dorsal surface of the (A) proximal and (B) distal phalanges of the great toe.

SUBJECT DIRECTIVE: *"Straighten out your big toe and hold it. Do not let me push it down."*

■ Grade 3/5: See Figure 2-84.

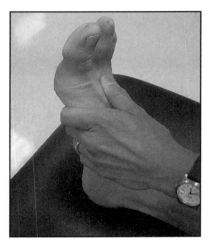

Figure 2-84. The subject is able to actively extend the great toe through the maximal range of motion without resistance.

■ Grade 2/5 is assigned for partial range of motion

GRADES 1/5 (TRACE) AND 0/5 (ZERO)

Subject position: Sitting or supine with both lower limbs extended and with the ankle in neutral.

Stabilization: The clinician stabilizes the foot and first metatarsal bone. See Figure 2-85.

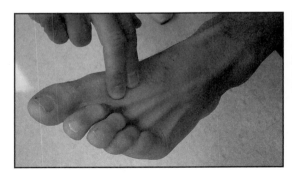

Figure 2-85. The extensor hallucis longus tendon is palpated on the dorsum of the foot lateral to the tibialis anterior tendon as it crosses the dorsum of the first metatarsal.

Grade 1/5 is assigned if the tendon movement is observed or palpated as the subject attempts to extend the great toe.

Points of interest: The strength of the extensor hallucis longus is assessed when suspecting L5 radiculopathy.

TOES II TO V

MTP FLEXION

ACTIVE RANGE OF MOTION

- 0 to 40 degrees

PRIME MOVERS

- Lumbricals

  □ Origin: Medial and adjacent sides of the flexor digitorum longus tendon to each lateral digit.

  □ Insertion: Medial aspect of the proximal phalanx and extensor hood of the 4 lateral toes.

  □ Innervation: Lateral plantar nerve (L5 to S2).

  □ Other actions: Extension of the PIP/DIP joints of the 4 lateral toes.

  □ Palpation site: Too deep to palpate.

SECONDARY MOVERS

- Dorsal and plantar interossei
- Flexor digiti minimi brevis
- Flexor digitorum brevis
- Flexor digitorum longus

GRADES 5/5 (NORMAL), 4/5 (GOOD), 3/5 (FAIR), AND 2/5 (POOR)

Subject position: Sitting or supine with both limbs maximaly extended and with the tested ankle/foot in neutral resting on a table.

Stabilization: The clinician stabilizes the lateral 4 metatarsal bones.

- Grades 5/5 and 4/5: See Figure 2-86.

Figure 2-86. Resistance is applied to the plantar surface of the metatarsophalangeal joints of the 4 lateral toes into metatarsophalangeal extension.

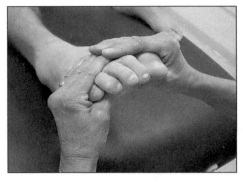

SUBJECT DIRECTIVE: *"Curl your toes over my fingers and hold it. Do not let me straighten them out."*

- Grade 3/5: See Figure 2-87.

Figure 2-87. A grade of 3/5 is assigned if the subject is able to flex the metatarsophalangeal joints but is unable to hold them in position with any resistance. A grade of 2/5 is assigned if the subject can only move the toes through partial range of motion.

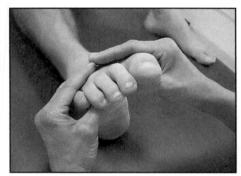

GRADE 1/5 (TRACE) AND 0/5 (ZERO)

A grade of 1/5 is assigned if the clinician observes/palpates the contractile activity but no toe motion occurs.

Points of interest: Weakness of the lumbricals can result in hammer toes and loss of the transverse arch of the foot.

DIP AND PIP FLEXION

ACTIVE RANGE OF MOTION

- 0 to 35 degrees (PIP)

- 0 to 65 degrees (DIP)

PRIME MOVERS

- Flexor digitorum brevis

  - Origin: Medial process of the calcaneal tuberosity.

  - Insertion: Tendon slips to the base of the middle phalanx of toes II to V.

  - Innervation: Medial plantar nerve (S1 to S2).

  - Other actions: Flexion of the MTP joints of the 4 lateral toes.

  - Palpation site: The tendons are palpable on the plantar surface of the proximal phalanx of toes II to V.

- Flexor digitorum longus

  - Origin: Middle two thirds of the posterior tibial shaft.

  - Insertion: Base of the distal phalanx of toes II to V.

  - Innervation: Tibial nerve (L5 to S2).

  - Other actions: Flexion of the MTP joints of the 4 lateral toes and slight plantar flexion of the ankle.

  - Palpation site: The tendons are palpable on the plantar surface of each middle phalanx of toes II to V.

SECONDARY MOVERS

- Quadratus plantae

GRADES 5/5 (NORMAL), 4/5 (GOOD), 3/5 (FAIR), AND 2/5 (POOR)

Subject position: Sitting or supine with both lower extremities maximaly extended and the ankle/foot in neutral resting on a table.

Stabilization: The clinician stabilizes the metatarsal bones of toes II to V.

- Grades 5/5 to 4/5: See Figure 2-88.

Figure 2-88. Resistance is applied under the plantar aspect of the proximal or distal phalanges, respectively, into extension.

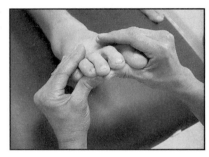

SUBJECT DIRECTIVE: *"Curl your toes over my fingers and hold it. Do not let me push them up."*

A grade of 3/5 is assigned if the subject is able to complete the range of motion but is unable to do so with resistance. A grade of 2/5 is assigned if the subject only completes partial range of motion.

GRADES 1/5 (TRACE) AND 0/5 (ZERO)

- Grades 1/5 to 0/5: See Figure 2-89.

Figure 2-89. The tendons of the flexor digitorum longus are palpated on the plantar surface of the middle phalanx of toes II to V.

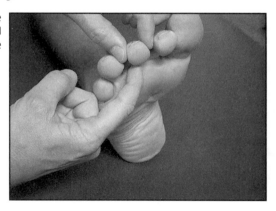

Points of interest: Weakness of the flexor digitorum longus may result in hyperpronation of the foot.

DIP AND PIP EXTENSION

ACTIVE RANGE OF MOTION

- 35 to 0 degrees (PIP)

- 65 to 0 degrees (DIP)

PRIME MOVERS

- Extensor digitorum brevis

  - Origin: Superolateral surface of the calcaneus.

  - Insertion: Lateral sides of the tendons of the extensor digitorum longus.

  - Innervation: Deep peroneal nerve (L5 to S1).

  - Other actions: Extension of the MTP joints of the 4 lateral toes.

  - Palpation site: The muscle belly is palpable on the dorsolateral surface of the foot.

- Extensor digitorum longus

  - Origin: Lateral condyle and lateral shaft of the tibia, proximal/anterior surface of the fibular shaft.

  - Insertion: Dorsal surface of the middle/distal phalanges of digits II to V.

  - Innervation: Deep peroneal nerve (L5 to S1).

  - Other actions: Extension of the MTP joints of the 4 lateral toes and slight dorsiflexion of the ankle joint.

  - Palpation site: Dorsolateral surface of the foot to each of the 4 lateral digits.

SECONDARY MOVERS

- None

Grades 5/5 (normal), 4/5 (good), 3/5 (fair), and 2/5 (poor)

Subject position: Sitting or supine with both lower extremities in maximal extension and the ankle/foot in neutral resting on a table.

Stabilization: The clinician stabilizes the metatarsal bones of toes II to V.

- Grades 5/5 to 4/5: See Figure 2-90.

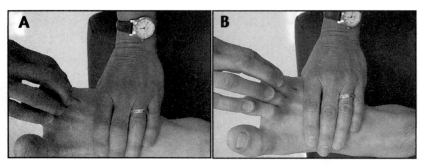

Figure 2-90. Resistance is applied to the dorsal surface of the (A) proximal and (B) distal phalanges into flexion to test PIP and DIP extension, respectively.

SUBJECT DIRECTIVE: *"Straighten your toes and hold it. Do not let me push them down."*

*A grade of 3/5 is assigned if the subject is able to complete the range of motion, but is unable to do so with resistance. A grade of 2/5 is assigned if the subject only completes partial range of motion.

GRADES 1/5 (TRACE) AND 0/5 (ZERO)

- Grades 1/5 and 0/5: See Figure 2-91.

Figure 2-91. The tendons of the extensor digitorum longus are palpated as they cross the dorsolateral surface of the foot as they course to each of the lateral 4 toes.

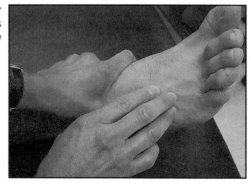

Appendices

Van Ost, L.
Cram Session in Manual Muscle Testing:
A Handbook for Students & Clinicians (pp. 179-188)
© 2012 SLACK Incorporated

APPENDIX A
KEY TO MANUAL MUSCLE GRADING

	MUSCLE ACTIVITY		KENDALL		DANIELS & WORTHINGHAM
No movement	No contraction felt in muscle	0	0	Zero	0	Zero
	Tendon is prominent and muscle contraction is palpable, no visible movement of tested body part	T	1	Trace	1	Trace
	GRAVITY MINIMIZED POSITION					
Test movement	Moves through partial range of motion	1	2–	Poor–	2–	Poor–
	Moves through complete range of motion	2	2	Poor	2	Poor
	ANTI-GRAVITY POSITION					
	Moves through partial range of motion	3	2+	Poor+	2+	Poor+
Test position	Gradual release from test position	4	3-	Fair–		
	Holds test position with no resistance	5	3	Fair	3	Fair
	Holds test position against slight resistance	6	3+	Fair+	3+	Fair+
	Holds test position against slight to moderate resistance	7	4–	Good–		
	Holds test position against moderate resistance	8	4	Good	4	Good
	Holds test position against moderate to strong resistance	9	4+	Good+		
	Holds test position against strong resistance	10	5	Normal	5	Normal

APPENDIX B
GENERAL PROCEDURE FOR MANUAL MUSCLE TESTING

- The subject should be positioned in a manner that ensures accurate testing and addresses comfort. The test position may need to be modified occasionally to minimize stress on other parts of the body.

- The subject should be positioned so that support is provided to the body as a whole so that the subject can focus on the body part being tested.

- The body part being tested should initially be placed in an antigravity position. If the muscles are too weak to function against gravity, the body part should be placed in a position in which gravity is minimized.

- The proximal aspect of the tested body part should be stabilized to decrease the compensatory action of other muscles that are not being tested.

- Resistance given during testing should be directly opposite to the "line of pull" of the muscles being tested.

- Resistance should be gradual and uniform, not sudden or "jerky." A long lever arm should be used unless contraindicated.

- Both sides of the body should be tested when appropriate to provide a comparison. This is especially important if there is a known injury/pathology of the tested side.

APPENDIX C
COMMONLY USED TERMS IN MANUAL MUSCLE TESTING

active resisted test: A muscle test in which the examiner gradually increases the amount of manual resistance until it reaches the maximal level the subject can tolerate and the movement stops. This type of testing is used infrequently because of the level of skill required to perform it accurately.

available range of motion: The full range of motion for that subject at the time of testing. Although it may not be normal, muscle grading is assigned within this range.

break test: A muscle test that is used to determine the maximal effort given by the subject when manual resistance is applied to the body part after it is placed at the end range position by the examiner. The subject is asked to "hold" the body part at the end of the available range of motion and not allow the examiner to "break" the hold with manual resistance. It is the most commonly used manual muscle testing procedure.

grading: The assignment of a word or numerical value based on an examiner's assessment of the strength or weakness of a muscle or muscle group. Grading values range from zero (0) to normal (5); zero denotes no muscle activity and five denotes normal activity, which is considered the best possible effort by the subject to the test.

resistance: The external force that opposes the test movement.

stabilization: The holding steady or holding down of a body part to ensure an accurate test of a muscle or muscle group.

substitution: A movement that results from one or more muscles attempting to compensate for the lack of strength in a muscle group or group of muscles.

test movement: The movement of a body part in a specified direction through a specific arc of motion.

test position: The position in which the body part is placed by the examiner and held by the subject.

weakness: Loss of movement of a body part as a result of a muscle not contracting sufficiently to move the body part through partial or full range of motion.

APPENDIX D
FACTORS THAT MAY CAUSE
INACCURATE MUSCLE TESTING

- The subject becomes distracted during testing.

- The subject experiences pain during testing.

- The subject is positioned improperly.

- The body part being tested is not adequately stabilized.

- Inability of the subject to understand the test requirements/commands as a result of poor comprehension or cultural and language barriers.

- The subject does not have the coordination to perform the test adequately.

- Inadequate understanding of basic anatomy/kinesiology by the clinician.

- Poor awareness of basic substitution patterns by the clinician.

- "Overgrading" or "undergrading" a muscle as a result of clinician inexperience.

- Inconsistency in timing, pressure, and positioning by the clinician.

- The use of gloves by the clinician may alter the ability to palpate a muscle contraction accurately.

- External devices or equipment in the environment may limit the clinician's ability to adequately test a body part.

BIBLIOGRAPHY

Amundsen LR, ed. *Muscle Strength Testing; Instrumented and Non-instrumented Systems*. New York, NY: Churchill Livingstone; 1990.

Basmajian JV, De Luca CJ. *Muscles Alive; Their Functions Revealed by Electromyography*. Baltimore, MD: Williams & Wilkins; 1985.

Beasley WC. Quantitative muscle testing: principles and applications to research and clinical services. *Arch Phys Med Rehab*. 1961;42:398–425.

Bernier J. *Quick Reference Dictionary for Athletic Training*. 2nd ed. Thorofare, NJ: SLACK Incorporated; 2005.

Bohannon RW. Make tests and break tests of elbow flexor muscle strength. *Phys Ther*. 1988;68:193–194.

Bohannon RW. Internal consistency of manual muscle testing scores. *Percept Mot Skills*. 1997;85:736–738.

Bohannon RW. Manual muscle testing: does it meet the standards of an adequate screening test? *Clin Rehabil*. 2005;19:662–667.

Clarkson HM. *Musculoskeletal Assessment. Joint Range of Motion and Manual Muscle Strength*. 2nd ed. Philadelphia, PA: Lippincott, Williams & Wilkins; 2000.

Cole JH, Furness AL, Twomey LT. *Muscles in Action. An Approach to Manual Muscle Testing*. New York, NY: Churchill Livingstone; 1988.

Cuthbert SC, Goodheart GJ. On the reliability and validity of manual muscle testing: a literature review. *Chiropr Osteopat*. 2007;15.

Cutter NC, Kevorkian CG., ed. *Handbook of Manual Muscle Testing*. New York, NY: McGraw-Hill; 1999.

Donatelli RA, Wooden MJ. *Orthopedic Physical Therapy*. 4th ed. St. Louis, MO: Churchill Livingstone; 2010.

Durfee WK, Iaizzo PA. *Rehabilitation and Muscle Testing: Encyclopedia of Medical Devices and Instrumentation*. 2nd ed. Hoboken, NJ: John Wiley & Sons; 2006.

Dutton M. *Orthopaedic Examination, Evaluation, and Intervention*. 2nd ed. Columbus, OH: McGraw-Hill; 2008.

Evans RC. *Illustrated Orthopedic Physical Assessment*. 3rd ed. St. Louis, Mo: Mosby; 2009.

Hansen JT. *Netter's Clinical Anatomy*. 2nd ed. Philadelphia, PA: Saunders; 2010.

Hislop HJ, Montgomery J. *Daniels and Worthingham's Muscle Testing: Techniques of Manual Examination*. 8th ed. St. Louis, MO: Saunders; 2007.

Hollinshead WH. *Textbook of Anatomy*. 3rd ed. Philadelphia, PA: Harper & Row; 1974.

Hoppenfeld S. *Physical Examination of the Spine and Extremities*. New York, NY: Appleton-Century-Crofts; 1976.

Iddings DM, Smith LK, Spencer WA. Muscle testing: part 2. Reliability in clinical use. *Phys Ther Rev*. 1961;41:249–256.

Jepsen JR, Laursen LH, Larsen AI, Hagert CG. Manual strength testing in 14 upper limb muscles; a study of inter-rater reliability. *Acta Orthop Scand*. 2004;75:442–448.

Kendall FP, McCreary EK, Provance PG, Rodgers MM, Romani WA. *Muscles: Testing and Function with Posture and Pain*. 5th ed. Philadelphia, PA: Lippincott, Williams & Wilkins; 2005.

Lehmkuhl LD, Smith LK. *Brunnstrom's Clinical Kinesiology*. 4th ed. Philadelphia, PA: F.A. Davis Company; 1983.

Lilienfeld AM, Jacobs BA, Willis M. A study of the reproducibility of muscle testing and certain other aspects of muscle scoring. *Phys Ther Rev*. 1954;34:279–289.

Lippert LS. *Clinical Kinesiology and Anatomy*. 4th ed. Philadelphia, Pa: F.A. Davis Company; 2006.

Lovett RW, Martin EG. Certain aspects of infantile paralysis with a description of a method of muscle testing. *JAMA*. 1916;66:729–733.

Lunsford BR, Perry J. The standing heel-raise test for ankle plantar flexion: criterion for normal. *Phys Ther*. 1995;75:694–698.

Magee DJ. *Physical Assessment*. 5th ed. St. Louis, MO: Saunders; 2008.

Moore KL, Dalley AF, Agur AMR. *Clinically Oriented Anatomy*. 6th ed. Baltimore, MD: Lippincott, Williams & Wilkins; 2009.

Mulroy SJ, Lassen KD, Chambers SH, Perry J. The ability of male and female clinicians to effectively test knee extension strength using manual muscle testing. *J Orthop Sports Phys Ther*. 1997;26:192–199.

Nicholas JA, Sapega A, Kraus H, Webb JN. Factors influencing manual muscle tests in physical therapy. *J Bone Joint Surgery Am*. 1978;60:186–190.

O'Sullivan SB, Schmitz TJ. *Physical Rehabilitation: Assessment and Treatment*. 3rd ed. Philadelphia, PA: F.A. Davis Company; 1994.

Palmer ML, Epler ME. *Fundamentals of Musculoskeletal Assessment Techniques*. 2nd ed. Philadelphia, PA: Lippincott-Raven; 1998.

Reese NB. *Muscle and Sensory Testing*. Philadelphia, PA: W.B. Saunders Company; 1999.

Reider B. *The Orthopaedic Physical Examination*. 2nd ed. Philadelphia, PA: Saunders; 2005.

Rothstein JM, Roy SH, Wolf SL. *The Rehabilitation Specialist's Handbook.* 2nd ed. Philadelphia, PA: F.A. Davis Company; 1998.

Sapega AA. Muscle performance evaluation in orthopedic practice. *J Bone Joint Surg.* 1990;72:1562–1574.

Schwartz S, Cohen ME, Herbison GJ, Shah A. Relationship between two measures of upper extremity strength: manual muscle test compared to hand-held myometry. *Arch Phys Med Rehabil.* 1992;73:1063–1068.

Sieg KW, Adams SP. *Illustrated Essentials of Musculoskeletal Anatomy.* 4th ed. Gainesville, FL: Megabooks; 2002.

Smidt GC, Rogers MW. Factors contributing to the regulation and clinical assessment of muscle strength. *Phys Ther.* 1982;62:1283–1289.

Van Ost L. *Cram Session in Goniometry: A Handbook for Student and Clinicians.* Thorofare, NJ: SLACK Incorporated; 2010.

Wadsworth CT, Krishnan R, Sear R, Harrold J, Nielsen DH. Intrarater reliability of manual muscle testing and hand-held dynamic muscle testing. *Phys Ther.* 1987;67:1342–1347.

Williams M. Manual muscle testing, development and current use. *Phys Ther Rev.* 1956;36:797–805.

Williams M, Stutzman L. Strength variation through the range of motion. *Phys Ther Rev.* 1959;39:145–152.

Wintz MM. Variations in current manual muscle testing. *Phys Ther Rev* 1959;39:466–475.

Zimny N, Kirk C. A comparison of methods of manual muscle testing. *Clin Manag Phys Ther.* 1987;7(2):6–11.

INDEX

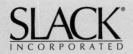